Shortcut to Orthopaedics

Shortcut to Orthopaedics

What's common and what's important for students and primary care physicians

Dr. Robert JR Perlau MD, FRCSC

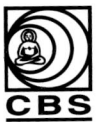

CBS Publishers & Distributors Pvt Ltd

New Delhi • Bengaluru • Chennai • Kochi • Kolkata • Mumbai
Hyderabad • Jharkhand • Nagpur • Patna • Pune • Uttarakhand

Shortcut to Orthopaedics

ISBN-13: 978-93-87085-91-6

CBS Reprint: 2018

Brush Education Inc.
www.brusheducation.ca
contact@brusheducation.ca

Photos: All photographs from the collection of the author unless otherwise specified as follows:iStockphoto.com: Figures 6.3 (kokopopsdave; 2732240), 8.1 and 21.3 (Getty Images; 51287292), 22.2 (nabari; 20524119), 25.3 (suemack; 6862392), 25.7 and 28.7 (StockPhotosArt; 28631260) 27.9 (johnnorth; 24627378) 28.8 (cteconsulting; 11504341). J. Kellen (Precision Orthotics): Figures 10.7, 14.3, 26.4, 27.2. G. Kiefer: Figures 19.5, 19.7, 19.10. 26.3, 26.7, 27.7. D. Malfair: Figures 2.20, 3.1, 3.9, 3.10. 3.11. 10.3, 13.2, 14.4, 14.5, 16.2, 23,5, 23,6, 26,5, 27,3, 27,5, 27,8. R. Perlau patients with permisson: Figures 7.1, 25.2, 28.1, 28.2

1. Orthopedics. I. Title.
RD731.P47 2015   C2015-901897-8   C2015-901898-6

Published by Satish Kumar Jain and Produced by Varun Jain for
CBS Publishers & Distributors Pvt Ltd
4819/XI Prahlad Street, 24 Ansari Road, Daryaganj, New Delhi 110 002, India.

Ph: 23289259, 23266861, 23266867   Fax: 011-23243014   Website: www.cbspd.com
e-mail: delhi@cbspd.com;
cbspubs@airtelmail.in.
Corporate Office: 204 FIE, Industrial Area, Patparganj, Delhi 110 092, India
Ph: 4934 4934   Fax: 4934 4935   e-mail: publishing@cbspd.com;
publicity@cbspd.com

Branches

- **Bengaluru:** Seema House 2975, 17th Cross, KR Road, Banasankari 2nd Stage, Bengaluru 560 070, Karnataka
  Ph: +91-80-26771678/79   Fax: +91-80-26771680   e-mail: bangalore@cbspd.com
- **Chennai:** 7, Subbaraya Street, Shenoy Nagar, Chennai 600 030, Tamil Nadu
  Ph: +91-44-26680620, 26681266   Fax: +91-44-42032115   e-mail: chennai@cbspd.com
- **Kochi:** Ashana House, 39/1904, AM Thomas Road, Valanjambalam, Ernakulam 682 016, Kochi, Kerala
  Ph: +91-484-4059061-65,67   Fax: +91-484-4059065   e-mail: kochi@cbspd.com
- **Kolkata:** 6/B, Ground Floor, Rameswar Shaw Road, Kolkata-700014 (West Bengal), India
  Ph: +91-33-2289-1126, 2289-1127, 2289-1128   e-mail: kolkata@cbspd.com
- **Mumbai:** 83-C, Dr E Moses Road, Worli, Mumbai-400018, Maharashtra
  Ph: +91-22-24902340/41   Fax: +91-22-24902342   e-mail: mumbai@cbspd.com

Representatives

- **Hyderabad** 0-9885175004   • **Jharkhand** 0-9811541605   • **Nagpur** 0-9021734563
- **Patna** 0-9334159340   • **Pune** 0-9623451994   • **Uttarakhand** 0-9716462459

Printed at Rashtriya Printer, Delhi, India

Contents

PART THREE   ORTHOPAEDIC TRAUMA IN CHILDREN

Acknowledgements

My interest in learning and teaching has been nurtured by the exemplary teachers and mentors I have worked with during my training and career in orthopaedics.

In Calgary: The late Dr. Gary Hughes who taught me "the enemy of good is better." Dr. Gerry Kiefer for his encouragement and kindness when I was a resident. Dr. Robert McMurtry who taught me the importance of being a "good doctor" as well as a "good surgeon."

In Boston: Dr. Michael Wilson who took this prairie boy under his wing, taught me how to write research papers, and helped me to navigate my orthopaedic fellowship.

In Red Deer: My orthopaedic and surgical colleagues who patiently supported me in my attempts to foster medical education.

Dr. Richard Buckley, Professor of Orthopaedic Trauma in Calgary, who gave me inspiration, leadership, and advice regarding orthopaedic education in Canada and beyond.

Perhaps, most of all, to my wife, Brenda (little Scoop), who helped me to keep the faith — in the project, and in myself.

Introduction

The purpose of writing this book came out of my experience teaching family medicine residents and medical students over 20 years of community orthopaedic practice.

The residents would routinely ask the same questions and would invariably be overwhelmed by the amount of information to learn on their orthopaedic rotation. The major problem for them was not weak prior teaching or aptitude, but that of perspective and relevance. What was really important for them to learn in orthopaedics and what would they see in practice?

This text is my attempt to organize the broad and increasingly sub-specialized field of orthopaedics into manageable units so the student, and ultimately the nonorthopaedic physician, will have a foundation to manage musculoskeletal problems.

This book is not intended to be all-inclusive in scope. The section on paediatric orthopaedics is limited to generally healthy children without underlying syndromes or conditions (such as cerebral palsy). Most of these disorders are managed by university-based paediatric orthopaedists. Hand injuries and disorders are excluded, as are cervical spine injuries and disorders: both are outside the usual scope of community-based orthopaedic surgery practice in Canada. However, the vast majority of common and important orthopaedic conditions seen in community practice are covered.

The material covered in this text should be familiar to all primary-care physicians starting out in practice in Canada. These foundational principles and skills will help physicians treat the majority of orthopaedic problems encountered with confidence.

DISCLAIMER

The publisher, authors, contributors, and editors bring substantial expertise to this reference and have made their best efforts to ensure it is useful, accurate, safe, and reliable.

Nonetheless, practitioners must always rely on their own experience, knowledge and judgement when consulting any of the information contained in this reference or employing it in patient care. When using any of this information, they should remain conscious of their responsibility for their own safety and the safety of others, and for the best interests of those in their care.

To the fullest extent of the law, neither the publishers, the authors, the contributors, nor the editors assume any liability for injury or damage to persons or property from any use of information or ideas contained in this reference.

Glossary

AC	acromio-clavicular	DVT	deep vein thrombosis
ACL	anterior cruciate ligament	ESR	erythrocyte sedimentation rate
ADL	activities of daily living		
AIIS	anterior inferior iliac spine	EUA	examination under anaesthetic
AIN	anterior interosseous nerve		
		FDL	flexor digitorum longus
AP	anterior posterior (X-ray)	FHL	flexor hallucis longus
ARDS	acute respiratory distress syndrome	GCT	giant cell tumour
		GI	gastrointestinal
ASIF	Association for the Study of Internal Fixation	GU	genitourinary
		HPF	high-powered field (microscope)
ASIS	anterior superior iliac spine	HTO	heterotopic ossification
		IM	intramuscular
ATLS	Advanced Trauma Life Support	INR	International Normalized Ratio
AVN	avascular necrosis		
BMI	body mass index	IP	interphalangeal
CBC	complete blood count	IV	intravenous
CC	coraco-clavicular	JIA	juvenile idiopathic arthritis
CHF	congestive heart failure		
CMC	carpal-metacarpal	JRA	juvenile rheumatoid arthritis
COPD	chronic obstructive pulmonary disease		
		LCL	lateral collateral ligament
CPPD	crystalline pyrophosphate disease	LMW	low molecular weight
		MC	metacarpal
CRF	chronic renal failure	MCL	medial collateral ligament
CT	computerized tomography	MI	myocardial infarct
CVT	congenital vertical talus	MP	metacarpal phalangeal
CXR	chest X-ray	MRI	magnetic resonance imaging
DDH	development dysplasia of the hip		
		MSK	musculoskeletal
DHS	dynamic hip screw	MT	metatarsal
DIC	diffuse intravascular coagulation	MTP	metatarsal phalangeal
		MVA	motor vehicle accident
DISI	dorsal intercalated segmental instability	N	normal
		NCS	nerve conduction studies
DJD	degenerative joint disease	NSAID	nonsteroidal anti-inflammatory drug
DRUJ	distal radial ulnar joint		
DSTR	distribution		

O/A	osteoarthritis
OCD	osteochondritis dissecans
ORIF	open reduction internal fixation
PA	posterior anterior (X-ray)
PIP	proximal interphalangeal
PMTO	proximal metatarsal osteotomy
PTB	patellar tendon bearing
PTE	pulmonary thrombo embolus
R/A	rheumatoid arthritis
R/O	rule out
ROM	range of motion
RSDS	reflex sympathetic dystrophy syndrome
Rx	treatment
SCFE	slipped capital femoral epiphysis
SI	sacroiliac
SLAC	scapholunate advanced collapse

SLAP	superior labral anterio posterior
SNAC	scaphoid nonunion advanced collapse
SPF	spastic peroneal flatfoot
TEV	talipes equino varus
TFCC	triangular fibrocartilage complex
TFN	trochanteric femoral nail
THR	total hip replacement
TKR	total knee replacement
T/L	thoracolumbar
TLSO	thoracolumbar sacral orthosis
UBC	unicameral bone cyst
U/S	ultrasound
WBC	white blood cell
WCB	workers' compensation board
XR	X-ray

PART ONE

BACKGROUND

1

Orthopaedics in Perspective

Being involved in medical training is always overwhelming, especially when you begin a new field of study and realize how much there is to learn. Orthopaedic surgery is no exception — it is a huge field spanning all age groups and affecting all parts of the body in the musculoskeletal (MSK) system.

All the various disease processes can affect the MSK system and enter into the differential diagnosis. Historically, traumatic and infectious disorders and their sequelae (such as polio or tuberculosis) have caused most of the pathology in orthopaedics. We can take a step back in time in orthopaedic care if we travel to the developing world today.[1] In the developed world, we still have trauma and its sequelae producing our caseloads, but degen-

---
Degenerative disorders dominate our elective practices.

---

erative disorders, rather than infection, now dominate our elective practices.

People are living longer and are healthier at older ages than they were a generation ago. Now, people's hips and knees are routinely replaced in order to maintain mobility, even though their parents may have been resigned to sit in a wheelchair because there were no other viable treatment options. The average age of hip-fracture patients continues to rise due to improved medical management of co-morbidities such as diabetes, heart disease, and lung disease.[2]

Medicine will never be free from infection and its sequelae, but primary osteomyelitis or septic arthritis is now uncommon. Today, infection presents in situations where immunity is somehow compromised or in the patient with an orthopaedic implant.

Fortunately, in orthopaedics, primary bone tumours are rare and death is uncommon. Metastatic pathological fractures can be fixated and radiated, with gratifying results for patients, and are rarely terminal events. There is, however, a significant one-year mortality rate in elderly hip-fracture patients (15%–25%) due to complications from the original injury.[3] Most of these patients die outside of hospital.

What specialists in this area do have to deal with is chronic disability. Almost every orthopaedic condition affects a person's mobility and ability to work or to pursue his or her vocation in

> Orthopaedic conditions cause minimal mortality but maximal chronic disability.

life. Recovery from elective orthopaedic surgery and from most fractures takes 3–6 months. Recovery from a fractured hip or multiple trauma takes at least one year and may never be complete. In addition, a healed fracture alone does not always equate with a successful outcome.

Patient expectations vary widely: work demands, activity levels, and hobbies all come into play and are of particular importance in orthopaedics. Young patients with high-energy traumatic injuries in particular need to be told as soon as possible that they may be unable to achieve their pre-injury levels of work or sport, even once the fracture is healed.

Outcomes are also affected by timely access to care. What is an appropriate wait time for hip replacement or fractured ankle surgery? When does an elective condition become urgent? What does urgent — or emergent — care mean? Ideally, most displaced fractures or dislocations, and most significant infections, should be treated within 12–24 hours. Minimally displaced fractures can be treated within 5–7 days, provided they have been well splinted. Elective orthopaedic surgeries should be performed within 3 months of surgical consultation. The longest wait, generally, is for the initial consultation, with patients often waiting up to 2 years.[4] The whole area of wait times in medical care has become a hot political issue for politicians and hospital administrators in recent years since public funding is involved. So-called "benchmarks for care" are being developed for health care delivery across jurisdictions.[5]

Energy Level and Age of the Patient

In my years of orthopaedic practice, I have found that two factors, more than any others, predict what pathology/injury will be found and what the likely outcome will be. The first is the age of the patient; the second is the amount of energy involved in the original injury.

First, the age of the patient predicts the weak link when force is applied to a joint or extremity. As the bones and joints develop, grow, mature, and then degenerate, one can predict where they will fail at each stage when a pathological force is applied. I have found this to be very useful clinically. A valgus blow to the lateral knee, for example, will cause a Salter II fracture of the distal femur in a 15-year-old, an MCL tear in a 25-year-old, and a lateral tibial plateau fracture in a 70-year-old. In non-traumatic conditions, age predicts patterns we see repeatedly: hypermobility joint issues in the young, overuse conditions in adults, and degenerative conditions in the older age group.

> The age of the patient and the amount of energy involved in the original injury predict the outcome.

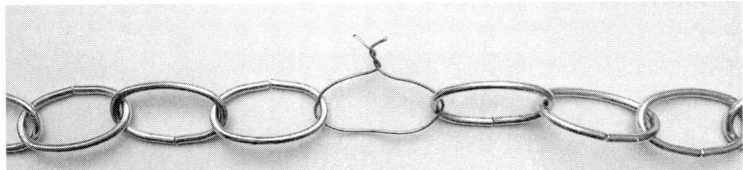

Figure 1.1 The age of the patient predicts the weak link in the joint or bone.

Second, the amount of energy involved in the trauma, or the sequelae of the trauma, significantly predicts the outcome. As the energy rises, the fracture becomes more fragmented, there is more soft tissue damage, and multiple body areas can be involved. These fractures are more difficult to fix initially, take longer to heal, and have more early and late complications. Even if you are seeing a patient years later with a post-traumatic degenerative condition, the amount of energy involved in the original accident can predict the outcome and potential reconstruction challenges. Orthopaedic histories may be brief, but one must get an idea of how much energy was involved in producing the injury.

In summary then, the conditions we see and the treatments we use in orthopaedic practice are evolving over time. Disability is a significant issue and patients are less tolerant of their limitations than previous generations. Finally, the energy level involved in the injury and the age of the patient will predict where the weak link around the bone and joint resides and what fracture pattern and outcome one will likely see.

REFERENCES
1. Foulkes WJR. *Orthopaedics overseas address* to annual *COA* meeting, Montreal, QC. 2005.
2. Leslie WD, O'Donnell S, Jean S, et al. Trends in hip fracture rates in Canada. *JAMA.* 2009;302(8):883–9.
3. Weller I, Wai EK, Jaglal S, et al. The effect of hospital type and surgical delay on mortality after surgery for hip fracture. *J Bone Joint Surg Br.* 2005;87-B(3):361–6. http://dx.doi. .g/10.1302/0301-620X.87B3.15300. Medline:15773647
4. Canadian Joint Registry Data Bulletin to Surgeons; 2008.
5. Sanmartin C, Berthelot JM, McIntosh CN. Determinants of unacceptable waiting times for specialized services in Canada. *Healthc Policy.* 2007;2(3):e140–54. Medline:19305710

2

Making a Diagnosis

The foundation of orthopaedic treatment, as in any medical discipline, is making the correct diagnosis. For non-orthopaedic-referring physicians, the major job is stabilizing the patient, making a diagnosis, and then communicating that information to the orthopaedic specialist in a clear and organized manner. Determining the urgency of the referral is also very important. Most orthopaedic surgeons will make time to see urgent referrals if the primary-care physician phones directly.

The orthopaedic history follows the general medical format but has a few specific nuances. It can be brief, but it should be focused. The orthopaedic physical exam should be well organized — it should flow: walking, standing, sitting, supine, prone. The tag line *look, feel, move, measure* applies to all parts of the MSK system. Usually, there is a normal, unaffected joint/limb to compare findings to when detecting abnormalities. There can be a great variation of "normal" from patient to patient in joint mobility and laxity.

> Physical exam for any MSK anatomic region: *look, feel, move, measure.*

Diagnostic imaging tests should be ordered logically — from simple to complex — and should be cost-effective, if possible. Magnetic resonance imaging (MRI) exams are over-requested by patients and family doctors and do not produce a faster referral to an orthopaedic surgeon. Many family doctors feel an orthopaedic surgeon will order an MRI anyway, so why not do something for the patient while he or she is waiting for orthopaedic consultation. This is not generally the case and in no way speeds the time to consultation. The following checklist will help in determining when an MRI is useful before referral.

CHECKLIST OF WHEN AN MRI IS USEFUL

MRI is very useful for
- complex soft tissue knee injuries (ligaments and menisci)
- complex sports-related shoulder injuries (more than the rotator cuff alone)
- complex wrist ligament disorders
- spinal conditions with nerve involvement
- soft tissue masses and tumours

MRI is not useful for
- simple osteoarthritis of any joint (actually better seen on plain X-rays!)
- degenerative knee arthritis/meniscal debris
- simple rotator cuff integrity (use ultrasound)
- fracture work (use plain X-rays or computerized tomography [CT] scan)

Plain X-rays are still the cornerstone of orthopaedic diagnosis and the primary-care physician must be able to communicate the patient's X-ray findings concisely to the orthopaedic specialist when referring a patient. Describing a plain X-ray is a vitally important skill and is not as easy as it sounds!

Some remarks about the general principles in orthopaedic history-taking, physical examination, and plain X-rays will be discussed first, followed by a more focused anatomic region-by-region discussion.

Orthopaedic History

The orthopaedic history should follow the normal format of any medical history: identification, chief complaint, history of present complaint, past medical history, social history, and family history. In the orthopaedic context, the following checklist is particularly useful.

CHECKLIST FOR ORTHOPAEDIC HISTORY

History of present illness
1. Age of patient:
   - *if traumatic:* Age predicts where the weak link may be present and, therefore, what injury pattern to expect.
   - *if atraumatic:* It broadly predicts what disorders are prevalent.

2. Symptom onset and trends:
   - *if traumatic:* The amount of energy involved in producing the injury is very important as it predicts initial outcomes and future complications.

- *if atraumatic:* precipitating events
- *trends*: worsening, stable, or improving

3. Aggravating and relieving factors:
   - Most MSK problems worsen with activities and improve with rest.
   - Some joints are quite specific: shoulder pain with overhead activities; knee pain with stair climbing.

4. Treatment thus far:
   - analgesics; NSAID; physiotherapy; Depo-Medrol injections; massage; MSK surgical procedures; walking aid needed

5. Occupation:
   - time off work; effect on work
   - handedness, if an upper-extremity problem

6. WCB-related problem?
   - This should be asked at the outset since it may be more complicated and affect outcomes.
   - for WCB cases: Documentation must be more complete; return to work time may be significantly longer.[1]

7. ADL intact:
   - basic activities: sleep, and pain at night?; walking distance and aid required?; stair climbing and kneeling; ability to dress oneself

8. Quality of life activities:
   - This varies greatly from patient to patient and in different age groups: a young high-performance athlete has different needs and expectations than a sedentary elderly patient.
   - Sports played and hobbies enjoyed by patients are very pertinent to the orthopaedic history.

Past medical history

1. Some co-morbidities definitely affect outcomes in orthopaedics and should be documented:
   - obesity, especially BMI greater than 35
   - obesity diabetes
   - obesity CRF
   - obesity coronary artery and peripheral vascular disease
   - obesity COPD
   - obesity cancer

2. Current medication list:
   - This is important and can often predict problems in the pre-op patient. Watch for use of Coumadin and for chronic narcotic analgesic use.

3. Adverse reactions:
   - Reaction to previous anaesthetics should be documented.

Social history
1. Cigarette smoking:
   - Always ask. Smoking negatively affects wound and bone healing[2] as well as anaesthetic risk.
   - Smokers tend to get out of bed earlier than non-smokers after surgery, to get outside to smoke, but this is the only (dubious) benefit.

2. Alcohol and illicit drug use:
   - Tricky to ask about and even harder to get a truthful answer, but they really do adversely affect outcomes, usually because compliance with treatment is so compromised.
   - Look for indirect clues to abuse, such as loss of driver's license (due to impaired driving), or analgesic requests by the patient "on the hour" when in hospital, in drug abusers.

Family history
Some family trends are seen in orthopaedics, but these are generally not as important as in some other disciplines. In paediatric orthopaedics, genetics plays a larger role. The following lists some family history considerations:
- *early osteoarthritis:* does run in families
- *rheumatoid arthritis:* does run in families
- *malignant hyperthermia:* rare, but does run in families; can be disastrous if missed

Physical Exam

The orthopaedic physical exam should be organized and should *flow naturally* regarding patient positioning: the sequence walk, stand, sit, supine, prone works comfortably for the patient. In orthopaedics, we have the advantage of dealing with paired appendages, so always *compare* the affected limb/joint to the normal (or less-affected) side. This is also helpful when ordering plain X-rays, particularly in children, when growth centres are present and can be confusing.

> Always compare the affected limb/joint to the normal (or less-affected) side.

Remember to include the joint *above* and the joint *below* in your examination (and on plain radiographs) as referred pain is common.

The pattern *look, feel, move, measure* can be used in any anatomic area in the MSK system:
- *look:* swelling; alignment; deformity; colour

- *feel:* effusion; crepitus; point of maximal tenderness (very important in diagnosis, especially in more superficial joints)
- *move:* active and passive range of motion (ROM); joint stability tests
- *measure:* ROM; leg lengths; muscle strength

Vascular Physical Exam

By convention, we do a neurovascular exam, for completeness, when applicable. Vascular problems are important in elective and traumatic conditions.

ELECTIVE CONDITIONS

Vascular compromise can predict future problems with wound and bone healing, particularly if the patient is a smoker. Diabetics and patients with chronic peripheral vascular conditions are at high risk. Look for signs of *chronic* vascular compromise: shiny, hairless skin; venous stasis; poor pulse; cool extremities.

TRAUMATIC CONDITIONS

An acute injury to the large vessels needs to be ruled out in certain high-risk injuries. Signs of a compartment syndrome may also be present.

High-risk injuries include the following:

- displaced supracondylar humeral fractures (usually in children)
- knee dislocations
- crush injuries (especially feet/lower leg and hands/forearms)
- fractures associated with burns

Here we are looking for signs of *acute* vascular compromise:

- *skin colour and temperature:* if pale/white and capillary refill greater than 2 seconds = ischemia; limb may feel cool
- *limb swollen/purple* with faster than normal capillary refill = venous engorgement (This is the more common scenario seen in trauma, as true acute ischemia is rare.)
- *pulse palpation* hard to detect if the limb is swollen; reassuring if present and strong; palpate radial and ulnar artery at the wrist; dorsalis pedis and post-tibial artery at the ankle

Look for other *signs of compartment syndrome.* **The five Ps: puffy** (very firm or hard muscle compartment); **pain; paraesthesia**, plus the last two, which are late = **pulseless** and **pallor**.

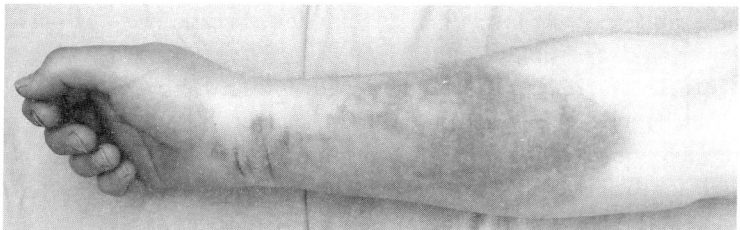

Figure 2.1 Compartment syndrome, right forearm

Neurological Physical Exam

The neurological orthopaedic exam is dictated by the clinical situation and a complete exam is not always required. One should always try to determine where the lesion is. As clinical experience grows, one will see certain patterns develop.

UPPER EXTREMITIES

CERVICAL SPINE DISORDERS

Cervical spine disorders can affect the nerve roots from C5 to T1 as well as the spinal cord itself. A detailed exam of dermatomes, myotomes, and reflexes, according to the list that follows, is indicated. Remember that everything flows from proximal to distal and reflexes follow myotomes.

- biceps reflex = C5/C6 elbow flexion
- triceps reflex = C6/C7 elbow extension
- brachioradialis reflex = C7/C8 wrist extension
- C8–T1 wrist/hand flexion

PERIPHERAL NERVE INJURIES

Peripheral nerve injuries are quite predictable with the following high-risk injuries:

- shoulder fracture/dislocations (axillary nerve)
- humeral shaft fractures (radial nerve)
- supracondylar elbow fractures (anterior interosseus nerve or ulnar nerve)
- wrist fracture/dislocations (median nerve)

Test for sensation and motor power in the autonomous zone for the nerve (no overlap of nerve function). The best tests are easy and painless for the patient to

Test in the *autonomous zones* as distally as possible.

perform (especially in trauma) and are done as distally as the nerve innervates as possible.

These simple tests can be done with minimal movement of the affected limb and little discomfort to the patient. Test the sensation in the autonomous zone and then determine if active movement is possible for the motor area listed as follows:

- *radial nerve:* sensation = dorsal thumb, index web space
  - · motor: Is thumb IP joint extension possible?

- *ulnar nerve:* sensation = volar tip of little finger
  - · motor = Can patient actively cross over index/long fingers?

- *median nerve:* sensation = volar tip of index finger
  - · motor = Can patient oppose thumb to little finger?

- *anterior interosseous nerve (AIN)*
  - · motor = Can patient flex IP of thumb and index finger together?
    - ~ = Round circle (normal) or a triangle (abnormal)?

- *axillary nerve:* sensory = boy scout patch of shoulder
  - · motor = Is deltoid abduction possible?

LOWER EXTREMITIES

Most neurologic lesions in the lower extremity originate in the lumbar spine and involve primarily the nerve roots and rarely the cauda equina.

Peripheral nerve lesions are much less common than those seen in the upper extremity. Exceptions would be an injury to the sciatic nerve (usually the common peroneal branch) from a posterior hip dislocation or an injury to the common peroneal nerve at the fibular head below the knee. These both produce weakness to foot eversion/dorsiflexion and numbness over the dorsum of the foot.

Nerve root examination follows the charts quite nicely and should include nerve tension signs. The most common disc lesions are seen at L4/L5 = L5 root (numb great toe; foot drop)

The most common peripheral nerve injury involves the sciatic nerve (peroneal branch) or peroneal nerve itself: result of both = a *foot drop.*

and L5/S1 = S1 root (numb sole/ lateral border of foot; weak plantar flexion; lost ankle reflex).

> The most common nerve root lesion is L5 or S1.

Cauda equina lesions can cause weakness and numbness at more proximal levels, including loss of knee reflex (L3/L4) and bowel/bladder dysfunction.

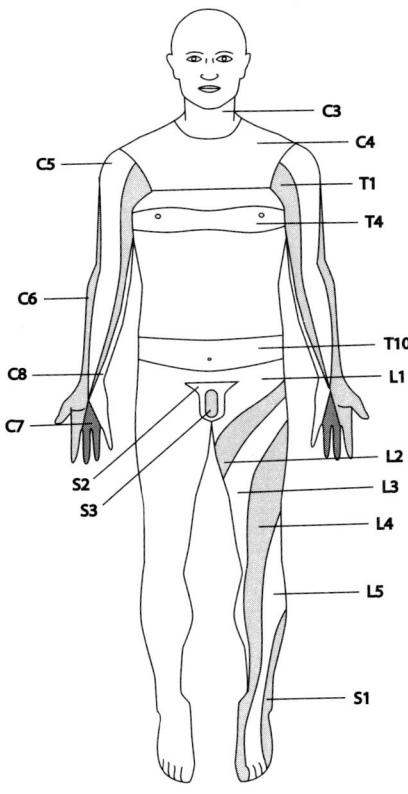

Figure 2.2 Schematic drawing of clinically relevant MSK dermatomes (upper and lower extremity)

Diagnostic Imaging: General Principles

In your history, always document the *exact* dates imaging tests were performed. This aids in being organized and precise, especially in medical–legal situations.

The imaging tests selected should follow a common-sense approach for patient inconvenience and expense of the test to the sys-

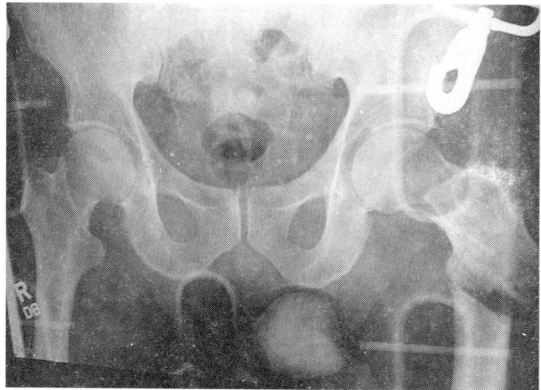

Figure 2.3 Apparent isolated left hip fracture

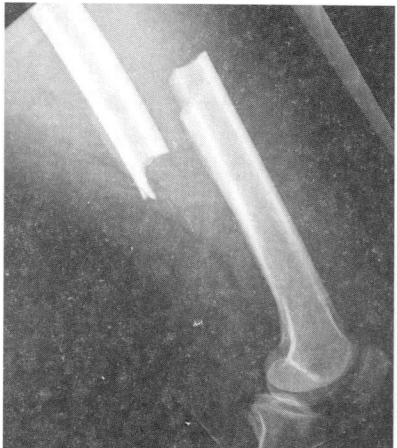

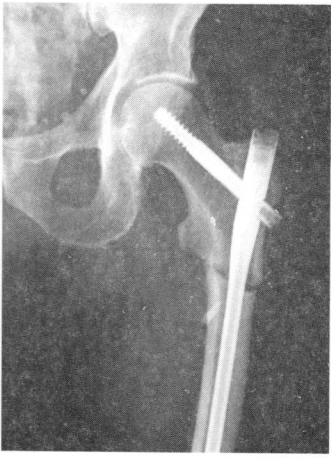

Figure 2.4 Missed ipsilateral left femoral shaft fracture

Figure 2.5 Fixation for both femur fractures

tem. Except in spinal conditions, 90% of the time plain X-rays alone are often enough, especially in fracture work and purely degenerative conditions. X-rays should be of good quality in at least two planes and should include the joint above and below the problem area.

Advanced scans are usually reserved for special circumstances:

- detailed bony anatomy around joints or the spine = CT scan

> Except in spinal conditions, plain X-rays alone are enough 90% of the time.

- soft tissue lesions: U/S or MRI
- nerve or spinal cord involvement = MRI
- multiple sites and bone activity = bone scan

Describing X-rays

Plain X-rays are the cornerstone of imaging in orthopaedics and cannot be underestimated. Properly describing an X-ray is a critical skill, especially when referring patients to orthopaedic surgeons.

DESCRIBING X-RAYS OF TRAUMA

In trauma cases, always try to convey the most significant abnormality first (malalignment, for example) and then comment completely on the other features. The summary of the X-ray should include the following:

- age of patient
- open or closed fracture
- displaced/non-displaced
- Location: which bone? where in bone (diaphysis; metaphysis; epiphysis/physis in children)?; very important to determine if the fracture is intra-articular
- Apposition/pattern: transverse, spiral, oblique, comminuted?; Remember that apposition of fragments is based on contact in two planes, AP and lateral XR (50% on AP + 50% on lateral XR = 25% apposition).
- Rotation: *Look* at relative thicknesses of cortices above/below the fracture; they should match.
- Alignment: *Measure* within 5–10 degrees. Always measure distal fragment relative to proximal. Measure the apex of the deformity location.

Some students find the acronym *LARA* helpful to remember these parameters.

Always describe the fracture or dislocation: distal fragment relative to the proximal.

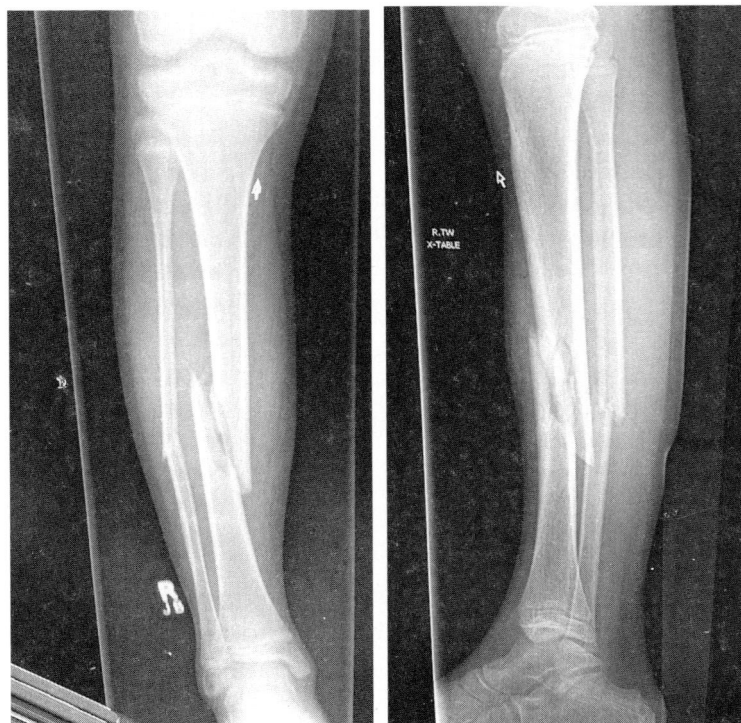

Figure 2.6 This is a 10-year-old boy with a closed, displaced, oblique fracture of the mid-shaft of the right tibia and fibula, with varus angulation of 15 degrees. The fracture is extra-articular, with 50% apposition of fragments, no malrotation, and good alignment in the lateral view.

CARDINAL RADIOGRAPHIC FEATURES OF ARTHRITIS (OSTEOARTHRITIS VERSUS INFLAMMATORY)

The second skill to acquire regarding plain X-rays is how to detect and describe the cardinal features of osteoarthritis (O/A) and how they differ from those seen in inflammatory arthritis (rheumatoid arthritis [R/A], etc.). Remember that the pathogenesis of these disorders is fundamentally different and this predicts what happens to the joint.[3]

Osteoarthritis is a degenerative condition where the bone/joint reacts to forces across abnormal joint surfaces: the joint tries to widen (osteophytes) and the bone becomes harder (subchondral sclerosis). Inflammatory arthritis is vascularly mediated and the bone becomes osteopenic and the joint erodes away.

	OSTEOARTHRITIS	RHEUMATOID ARTHRITIS
Joint space narrowing	• asymmetrical	• symmetrical
Bone density	• subchondral sclerosis • osteophytes	• osteopenia • no osteophytes
Cysts	• subchondral	• peri-articular erosions
Deformities	• joint collapse	• joint laxity/sublux

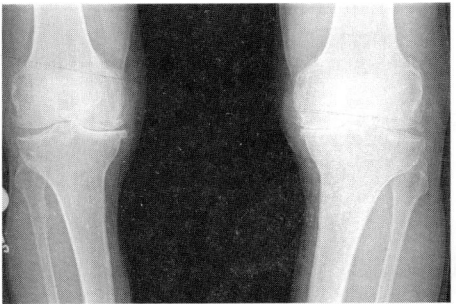

Figure 2.7 X-ray showing severe bilateral knee osteoarthritis

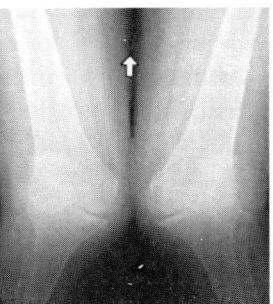

Figure 2.8 X-ray showing valgus joint laxity and erosions from severe rheumatoid arthritis

Region-by-Region Overview

Knee

Overall, the knee is perhaps the most common joint consulted upon by orthopaedic surgeons. In the younger age group, symptoms of instability predominate; in the older age group, stiffness predominates.

HISTORY

Obtain a detailed history of how the knee was injured, the treatment to date, and the investigations undertaken. Ask about the following:

- locking: when? for how long?
- instability: when? what activities?
- ADL: stairs? kneeling? stiff after sitting?
- need a cane or brace?
- walk or run? how far?
- analgesic use? night pain?

PHYSICAL EXAM

GAIT/ALIGNMENT/ROM

It is very important to evaluate the alignment of the knee when standing and walking. Weight bearing makes all the difference. Feel the joint while moving the knee, and measure the range of motion.

SPECIFIC TESTS FOR LIGAMENT LAXITY

All tests should compare the affected knee to the unaffected knee as people vary greatly in their ligamentous laxity. Be gentle, as only a small movement is required: you are looking for the amount of translation and the end-point feel.

MCL/LCL

For an MCL/LCL test, gently flex the knee and apply a valgus and varus force. Flexing the knee 10 degrees is important to avoid tightening the posterior knee capsule, which may produce a false impression of stability.

ACL TESTS

ACL tests are well described in many texts (anterior drawer; Lachman; pivot shift). Because it is easiest on the patient, the Lachman test is the best. Stand on the *same side* of the patient as the injured knee, as rotation is important, and flex the knee gently.

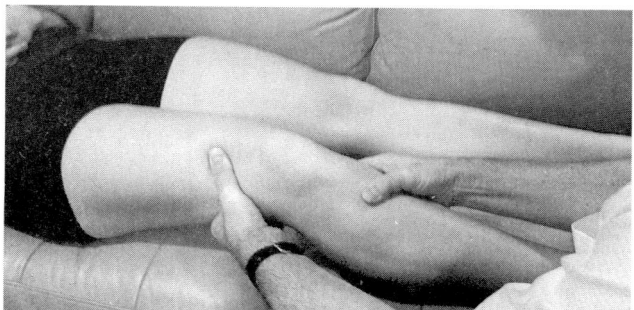

Figure 2.9 Lachman test: Feel for amount of translation and firmness of the endpoint; compare to the opposite normal knee.

MENISCAL TESTS

Meniscal tests include McMurray's test, Apley's test, and the joint line tenderness test. Be gentle: McMurray's test, in particular, can be painful for patients. A good history, coupled with joint line tenderness, is enough to clinch the diagnosis.

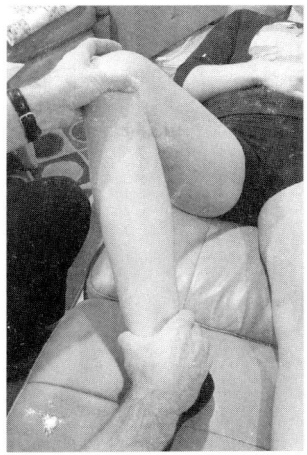

Figure 2.10 McMurray's test: Feel for painful clicking with your thumb on joint line while gently flexing and extending knee.

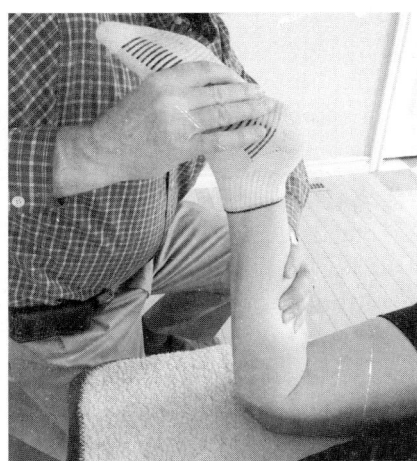

Figure 2.11 Apley's test: Compress and rotate for meniscal tears; distract and rotate for ligament tears.

KNEE IMAGING

Plain X-rays should be done with weight bearing if alignment or arthritis is an issue. Ultrasound is useful if a Baker's cyst is present.

An MRI is useful for detecting meniscal or ligamentous pathology and for tumours. However, it is grossly overused in the degenerative knee and is no better at diagnosing arthritis than plain X-rays. An MRI should be limited to the younger knee with soft tissue injuries where the diagnosis is still inconclusive after both physical exam and plain X-ray, and to knee patients requiring a tumour workup.

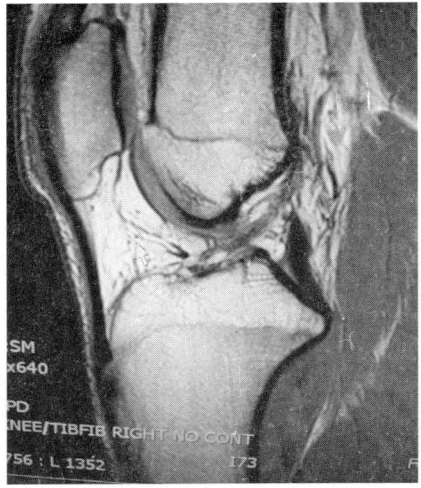

Figure 2.12 MRI knee with ACL injury (A normal ACL should be black and cord-like.)

Shoulder

The shoulder is the most common site of complaints in the upper extremity, in patients of all ages. Like the knee, young people tend to have problems with instability and older people with stiffness and weakness.

HISTORY

Age of the patient is quite predictive for the expected pathology in the shoulder: traumatic/instability issues in young people and degenerative arthritis and rotator cuff issues in older patients. Ask about the following:

- onset and trends
- details of instability feeling (arm position)
- analgesic use; pain at night?
- ADL intact (especially overhead activities and dressing)
- Rx to date (physio? Depo-Medrol?)

PHYSICAL EXAM

- *look:* muscle atrophy; proximal biceps rupture?
- *feel:* point tenderness; AC joint; joint crepitus?
- *move:* active and passive ROM (often differ)
  - · flex; extend; abduction; E.R.; internal rotation; elevation
  - · signs of impingement?
- *measure:* ROM, especially elevation

ROTATOR CUFF TESTS

- Grade on a scale of 0–5, where 0 = no muscle activity and 5 = normal strength.

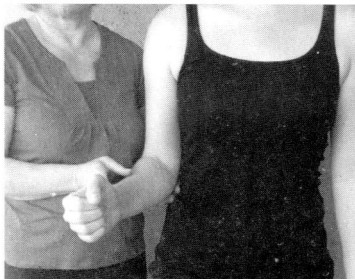

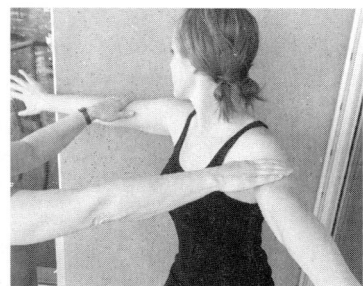

Figure 2.13 Infraspinatus test: resisted external rotation

Figure 2.14 Supraspinatus test: resisted abduction with internal rotation

INSTABILITY TESTS

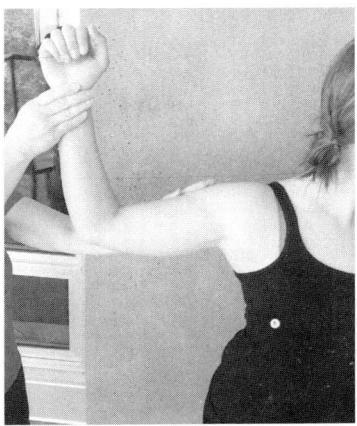

Figure 2.15 Shoulder: anterior instability apprehension test

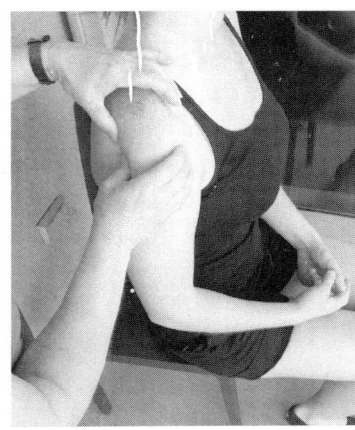

Figure 2.16 Passive subluxation test

SHOULDER IMAGING

Three plain X-ray views should be ordered routinely: AP, oblique, and trans-scapular lateral. Look at both the AC joint complex (for impingement) and the glenohumeral joint area (for osteoarthritis).

Ultrasound is an excellent and cost-effective way of detecting rotator cuff tears and whether they are partial- or full-thickness in nature.

A CT scan is very useful in complex fractures around the shoulder.

An MRI/arthrogram will show all the soft tissue features of the shoulder and is very useful for athletes (and also in usual situations such as tumours, infection, and AVN). In the older patient with a degenerative shoulder/cuff tear, an MRI is probably not necessary.

Hip/Low Back

The hip and low back should be examined together since there is so much overlap in symptoms (especially in the older age group). Referred pain from the spine into the hips and legs is a real concern.

HISTORY

The age of the patient is predictive of pathology in this area. Hip pathology is rare in young people (without childhood conditions) but very common in older adults. Lumbar disc disease can begin in young adulthood and persists into old age as degenerative changes develop in the spine (spinal stenosis). Ask about the following:

- onset and trends; back pain or leg pain dominant?
- site of pain: hip = groin or buttock?
- worse if walking? how far? coughing? night?
- better if standing, or must sit?
- numbness or weakness in legs?
- ADL: put on shoes/socks? cane needed?

PHYSICAL EXAM

Be organized with your exam:

- *walk/gait:* Trendelenburg?
- *stand:* L-spine ROM; alignment of spine/legs
- *sit:* leg lengths/hip rotation/neuro exam
- *supine:* hip/knee ROM; leg lengths; nerve tension tests/SI joints
- *prone:* hip extension; femoral stretch test; rectal?

The first motion lost in hip arthritis is internal rotation, so look for this in the sitting and supine position. Also look for flexion/abduction/external rotation contractures in the more advanced arthritic hip.

Leg length shortening is common in hip arthritis on the affected side and should be measured at the knee level both seated (with patient's buttocks against the chair back) and supine (from ASIS to medial malleolus).

Nerve tension signs (for sciatic nerve) can be done both seated and supine. Seated is more comfortable for the patient (and useful in dubious cases of sciatica).

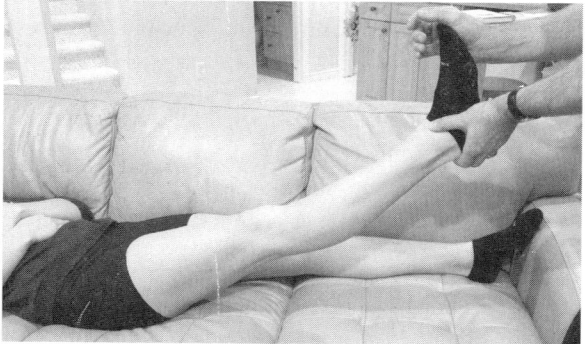

Figure 2.17 Straight leg raise for sciatic nerve tension

HIP/LOW BACK IMAGING

Plain X-rays should show the AP pelvis (a great screening test as shows both hips, SI joints, and lower lumbar spine). For the lumbar spine, get AP and lateral views. An AP/lateral hip X-ray is also useful.

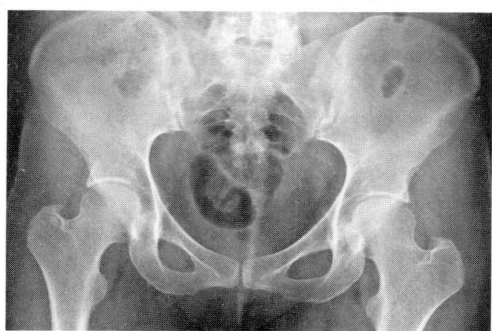

Figure 2.18 AP pelvis X-ray: great screening test for hips and lumbar spine

A CT scan is a good screening technique for lumbar disc disease or stenosis, as well as fractures.

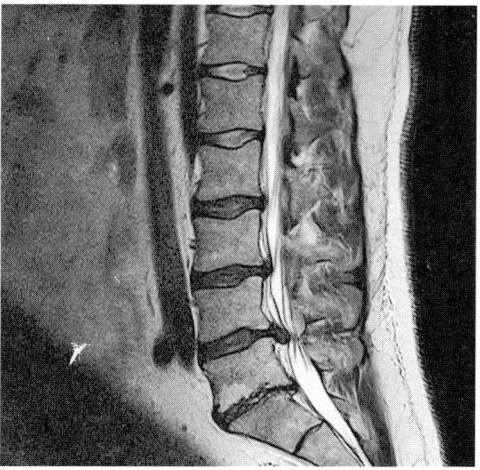

Figure 2.19 MRI of lumbar disc herniation

An MRI is best for showing neural elements in the spine. It is also good for infection versus tumour versus AVN.

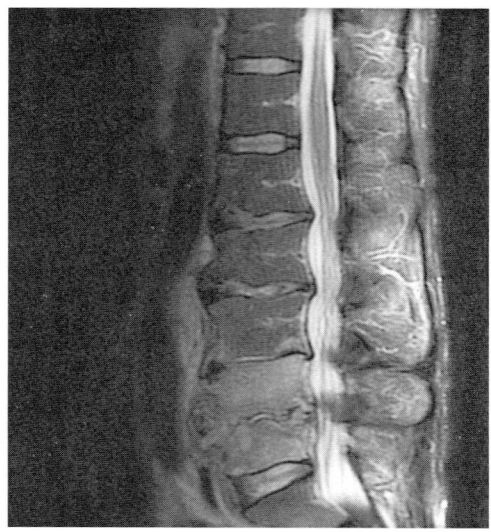

Figure 2.20 MRI of spinal infection (Note: Infection crosses disc space.)

Wrist/Elbow

Most of the conditions in the wrist/elbow region develop because of previous trauma or from repetitive strain and overuse. Obviously, then, handedness and work history are very relevant. Many of these patients are involved with the WCB, which may complicate their recovery.

Rheumatoid arthritis can greatly affect the hand, wrist, and elbow, often producing rather horrendous deformities.

HISTORY

Ask about the following:

- age
- onset and trends
- exact site of pain (This is quite revealing diagnostically.)
- aggravating and relieving factors
- work and effect on ADL
- patterns: stiff and weak versus sharp pain/clicking; radial versus ulnar wrist pain

- numbness (common, as median and ulnar nerves are very vulnerable)
- Rx to date

PHYSICAL EXAM

Always compare findings to the normal, opposite limb. The anatomy of the various joints is very superficial, so one can be quite specific in localizing the site of the problem by physical examination.

- *look:* joint swelling (soft tissue or bony); deformities (especially in rheumatoid arthritis)
- *feel:* seek out point of maximal tenderness (very diagnostic as joints are superficial); synovitis? crepitus? pressure over median, ulnar nerve provocation test; generalized ligamentous laxity?
- *move/measure:* ROM wrist and elbow; finger excursion (wrist supination and dorsiflexion usually lost first)
  · grip strength (percentage of normal)
  · instability tests: DRUJ wrist; collaterals elbow

WRIST/ELBOW IMAGING

The following plain X-rays are useful:

- Posterior anterior (PA); lateral wrist; scaphoid views
- AP; lateral elbow (Look for smooth equidistant joint spaces around all bones within the carpus.)

A CT scan is useful in scaphoid nonunions and fracture work.

Nerve conduction studies are useful in detecting median and ulnar nerve compression.

An MRI/arthrogram, with or without contrast, is useful for AVN, subtle ligament, and TFCC tears in the wrist.

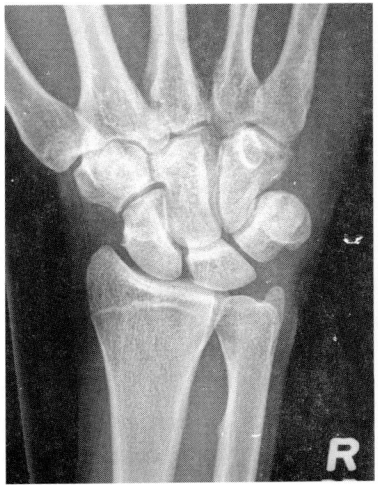

Figure 2.21 Normal PA wrist X-ray

Foot/Ankle

The foot/ankle area is a very common site for chronic pain without bony abnormalities ever being present. Heel pain, arch pain, and forefoot pain are examples of chronic soft-tissue-related pain. However, one must first rule out bone and joint disorders. These are often posttraumatic and degenerative in nature.

Diabetics can have horrendous problems with their feet, as can those with rheumatoid arthritis.

Pay particular attention to the peripheral vascular exam and neurological status since they greatly affect patient outcomes.

HISTORY

Ask about the following:

- site of pain; onset; trends
- unstable versus stiff/swollen
- worse on uneven ground/inclines?
- ADL intact?
- footwear problems?
- Rx to date (orthotics? braces?)

PHYSICAL EXAM

- *look:* Several areas yield diagnostic information:
  - shoes (wear patterns)
  - gait (N and heel and toe walking)
  - malalignment? hind-foot (varus/valgus); forefoot (great toe/ lesser toes)
- *feel:* Elicit the point of maximal tenderness (joints quite superficial); generalized ligamentous laxity?
- *move/measure:* ROM; instability tests for ankle

FOOT/ANKLE IMAGING

Plain X-rays of three views, preferably standing, will be useful.

A CT scan is quite useful if it shows bony detail, fractures, and the exact site of joint arthritis involvement. An MRI showing nerve or soft tissue disorders, tumours, and infection will also be useful.

In conclusion, orthopaedic conditions can be predictably diagnosed using a focused history and physical exam. Remember to use the unaffected joint or extremity to compare with whenever possible. Be organized in your physical exam and use *look, feel, move,* and *measure* as a general guide.

Plain X-rays are usually required as part of the orthopaedic exam, even in primary care. Describing the X-rays, particularly in trauma, is a very important skill to develop when referring patients to orthopaedic surgeons. More detailed diagnostic imaging should be reserved for specific indications only.

REFERENCES

1. Brauer CA, Manns BJ, Ko M, et al. An economic evaluation of operative compared with nonoperative management of displaced intra-articular calcaneal fractures. *J Bone Joint Surg Am.* 2005;87(12):2741–9. http://dx.doi.org/10.2106/JBJS.E.00166. Medline:16322625

2. Bender D, Jefferson-Keil T, Biglari B, et al. Cigarette smoking and its impact on fracture healing. *Trauma.* 2014;16(1):18–22

3. Klippel JH, editor. Pathogenesis of rheumatoid arthritis and osteoarthritis. *Primer on the Rheumatic Diseases.* 13th ed. Springer; 2008. p. 122–32.

Overview of Urgent Orthopaedic Conditions

Several situations require urgent orthopaedic care and a timely trip to the emergency department. Primary-care diagnosis and stabilization are necessary before referral, sometimes urgently, to the orthopaedic specialist. These situations, dealt with in this chapter, include the following:

1. multiply injured patient
2. open fractures
3. closed fractures
4. dislocations
5. limb pain: out of control
6. acutely swollen joint
7. soft tissue infections
8. acute back pain
9. child with a limp

Multiply Injured Patient

Primary-care doctors working in rural practice settings or any busy city emergency department will eventually be faced with the multiply injured patient. This is an extremely stressful situation for everyone involved because of the chaos that can ensue. The introduction of ATLS training courses and protocols has greatly improved the care of these patients in the emergency department.[1] These patients need to be stabilized and then transferred to secondary or tertiary hospitals as soon as possible.

Orthopaedic involvement follows the "life before limb" dictum. Once the ABCs have been dealt with and the patient has been stabilized, attention is then directed to the MSK system.

Although orthopaedic injuries are important, to keep things in perspective, remember that when dealing with multiple trauma, they are far down the list. The orthopaedic approach, in multiple trauma, should be prioritized.

> Remember: "life before limb" and "A B C D E F (is for fractures)."

1. Cover any open wounds (saline gauze).
2. Realign and splint any obviously crooked limbs.
3. Maintain spinal precautions until cleared radiographically: C-, T-, and L-spine (particularly important if patient was knocked unconscious or has a persistent decrease in consciousness and cannot protect their own spine).
4. Examine every joint/limb (for gross instability/deformity/pain); then order X-rays on suspect areas.
5. Perform cursory neurovascular exam on all four limbs.

Standard X-rays to order (at a minimum):

- CXR; AP pelvis; C-spine to T1
- AP and lateral X-ray of every clinically suspected area

General order of orthopaedic surgical treatment:

1. External fixation of unstable pelvic fractures: hours.
2. Wash out open wounds; stabilize associated fractures/dislocations: hours.
3. Fix femoral shaft and tibial shaft fractures (decrease ARDS): 12–24 hours.
4. ORIF remaining fractures (proximal, then distal) and spine: 24–96 hours.

These patients need to be stabilized and sent out of the primary-care setting as soon as possible. Once at the definitive treatment centre, the goal is to get the patient out of the recumbent position and upright as soon as possible in order to decrease sepsis, ARDS, and thrombosis.[2]

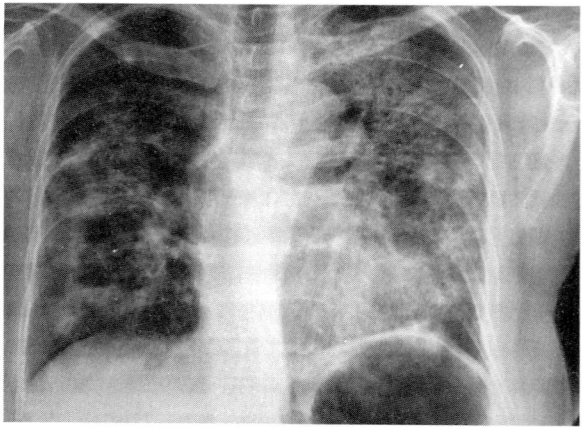

Figure 3.1 CXR demonstrating ARDS

Open Fractures

Open fractures imply high-energy injuries, with damage to the soft tissues, as well as to the underlying bone. They predictably occur in locations where there is little soft tissue coverage (tibial shaft; proximal ulna; hand and foot crush injuries) and from within/without at the apex of severely angulated fractures (medial ankle in ankle fracture/dislocation; volar forearm in severe dorsally angulated wrist fracture).

> Open fractures need to be definitively debrided in the O.R. within 6 hours.

These orthopaedic emergencies need to be debrided definitively in the O.R. within the "golden period" of 6 hours. Care in the emergency department is also important.

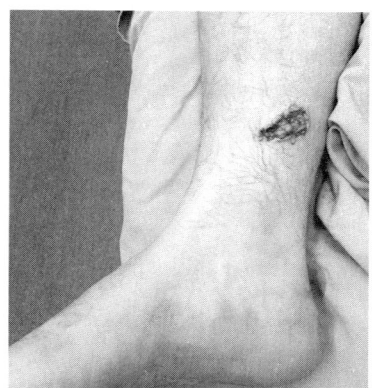

Figure 3.2 Grade II open fracture of distal tibia

THE PATIENT

- ABCs; intravenous (IV) access
- Start IV antibiotics (see following page).
- Check tetanus immune status.

THE LIMB

- Measure and sketch the location of the wound.
- Remove only large bits of detritus from the wound (glass, twigs, etc.).
- Cover with a saline gauze.
- Realign; splint the extremity.
- Check neurovascular exam.
- X-ray in two planes.

ANTIBIOTICS

The choice of IV antibiotics depends on the severity, or grade, of the open fracture. This system is based on the amount of energy involved in producing the open fracture, which is correlated in turn with the size of the open wound (Gustilo[3]). This system is widely used and quite predictive for complication rates and outcomes:

Grade I: wound less than 1 cm

Grade II: wound 1–9 cm

Grade III-A: wound 10 cm or larger that can be closed

Grade III-B: wound 10 cm or larger, flap needed for closure

Grade III-C: wound 10 cm or larger with vascular injury as well

Generally:

- *For Grade I and II open fractures*: IV Cefazolin is used (gram + organisms).
- *For Grade III open fractures:* Add gram negative +/- anaerobic coverage (aminoglycoside or a third-generation cephalosporin +/− clindamycin/metronidazole).
- *For really dirty wounds*: Add Penicillin G for *Clostridium perfringes*.

The antibiotics should be continued for 48 hours and then reassessed.

Closed Fractures

Primary-care physicians will be called to the emergency department on a regular basis to see patients of all age groups with closed fractures. The type of fracture seen in the community setting is predictable, as shown in the following list of common fracture patterns:

DEMOGRAPHIC PATTERNS OF COMMON FRACTURES

In the elderly

- hip fractures: These present on a daily basis in a busy hospital, regardless of the weather, since most of these fractures occur indoors and at home.
- wrist fractures: These are also common, as are impacted proximal humerus fractures.

In inclement, slippery weather

- fractured wrists and ankles in adults

Sports related

- knee ligament blowouts from skiing and hockey
- wrist and forearm fractures from snowboarding
- ankle and tibial fractures from soccer
- AC joint/clavicle fractures from cycling
- forearm and elbow fractures in children from trampolines and climbing

Alcohol related

- bad fractures from falls, often present days later (when sober)

The general treatment of all these fractures is the same: stabilize the patient first; then diagnose and splint the fracture. Any obviously crooked limb should be realigned and splinted before transfer. The fracture does not have to be reduced, only realigned to improve the circulation of the extremity and prevent skin breakdown over the apex of the deformity.

> Any obviously crooked limb should be realigned and splinted prior to transfer.

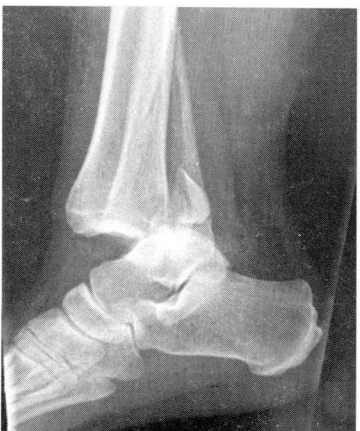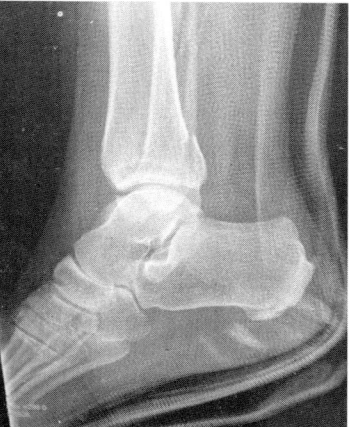

Figure 3.3 This unstable ankle injury was nicely realigned before transfer.

Make sure good-quality X-rays are ordered in two planes and the joint above and below the fracture is included, whenever clinically relevant.

The *ideal* timing for definitive fracture treatment varies depending on the neurovascular situation, the amount of residual displacement after realignment, and the status of the soft tissues.[4] General guidelines for the timing of fracture treatment are as follows:

TIMETABLE OF FRACTURE TREATMENT	
• fractures with neurovascular compromise	• within 6 hours
• any irreducible or significantly malaligned fracture	• within 12–24 hours
• hip fractures	• within 48 hours ideally
• femoral shaft fractures	• within 24 hours
• well-reduced fractures	• 24–96 hours (certainly no later than 2 weeks, as healing has already begun)

Dislocations

Dislocations can occur with or without an associated fracture and are most common in younger adults with good bone where the weak spot around the joint is through the capsule and ligaments rather than the bone itself. Pure dislocations are, therefore, rare in children and in the elderly.

With enough force and energy, any joint can dislocate (higher energy often produces associated fracture fragments), but these are the common sites:

- *shoulder:* occasionally with a greater tuberosity fracture
- *patellar:* always laterally; young patients, mostly girls; lax ligaments
- *ankle:* often with fracture; all ages; often subluxed only

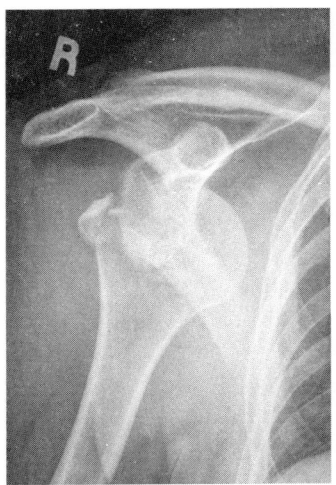

Figure 3.4 Anterior shoulder dislocation (with small greater tuberosity fracture)

- *hip:* common if THR present (rare, high energy with fractured acetabulum, if no THR)
- *elbow:* pure dislocation, or with fracture; high-energy injury
- *fingers/toes:* dislocation alone, or look for associated fractures

These common dislocations can be treated with closed reduction and splinting in the emergency department. Adequate muscle relaxation/analgesia and a backup person for airway maintenance are the keys to a successful reduction. (See Chapter 28 for more on closed-reduction techniques.)

Good-quality X-rays should be obtained before the reduction to ensure there is nothing unusual present to block or complicate the reduction. A large fracture fragment or a previously loose THR component, for example, would lead to complications. Postreduction X-rays should then confirm that success was obtained. If successful, referral to the orthopaedics clinic can be semi-elective. If unsuccessful, definitive reduction should occur within 12–24 hours and should be done in the O.R. under general anaesthetic.

Limb Pain: Out of Control

Patients sometimes present to the emergency department, often in the postoperative period, with significant and increasing extremity pain. Often, the operating surgeon is unavailable for consultation at the time.

Most of these cases are caused by swelling postfracture reduction or postsurgery. No fracture reduction is so precarious that the bandage or cast cannot be opened or removed. Bandages should be opened right to the skin; casts should be univalved or bivalved after an X-ray has been taken. Try to univalve the cast first on the non-buttressing side; for example, on the volar side in a typical dorsally angulated Colles' fracture. If this is ineffective, bivalve the cast or remove it completely.

Most patients will experience almost immediate relief of pain and improvement in skin colour of the fingers or toes. If this does not occur, consider other causes:

- *early wound infections:* obvious once bandage or cast is removed: localized wound redness, swelling, and drainage typical
  - · Treat aggressively with dressing changes and antibiotics (particularly if underlying implant is present).

- *deep vein thrombosis* (DVT): usually in the lower limb; slower onset; swelling persists regardless of dependent position of limb; look for risk factors in patient
  - Order venous Doppler test.

- *true compartment syndrome:* very serious, but uncommon: seen in high-energy trauma and certain anatomic areas; usually forearm or lower leg (although any muscle compartment can be involved)[5]

HIGH-RISK INJURIES FOR COMPARTMENT SYNDROME
- fracture/dislocation around elbow and knee
- high-energy closed tibial fractures
- high-energy closed forearm fractures
- crush injuries (especially feet)
- extremity burns
- revascularization of limb (embolectomy, etc.)
- drug overdose/unconscious patient (pressure on muscle compartment greater than 6 hours)

COMPARTMENT SYNDROME DIAGNOSIS CHECKLIST
- high-risk injury
- five Ps
  - **pain**, increases on passive movement of fingers or toes (quite specific test)
  - **puffy** compartment: should be firm, or hard
  - **paraesthesia; pulseless; pallor** (all late findings)
- compartment pressure testing greater than 30 mm Hg
- Use the compartment pressure-testing device, if available, but if in doubt, send patient for a fasciotomy.

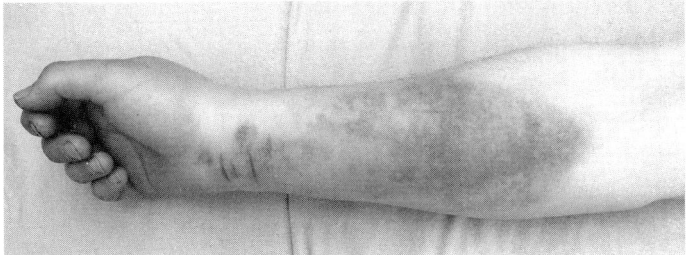

Figure 3.5 Compartment syndrome of right forearm

Definitive treatment is an open fasciotomy of all potential compartments involved. This should ideally be done within 6 hours. Patients often need a skin graft to close the wound.

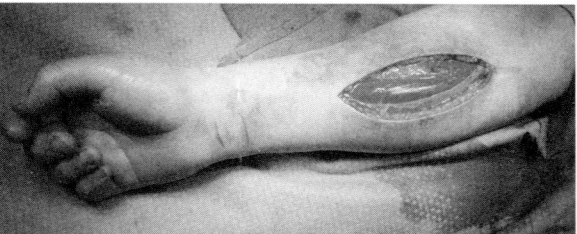

Figure 3.6 Fasciotomy of right forearm

Dramatic compartment syndromes are usually seen in the context of high-energy trauma, are obvious, and are rarely missed. Occasionally, however, subtle compartment syndromes are missed and present months or years later; for example, progressive claw toe formation after a tibial shaft fracture treated with closed nailing.

In summary, one must be vigilant. When in doubt, call the orthopaedic surgeon and he or she can decide if a fasciotomy is indicated.

Acutely Swollen Joint

Patients often present to the emergency department with an acutely swollen and painful joint. The knee joint is most often involved, but any joint, except the hip (because swelling is masked by its deep anatomy), can present in this fashion. All age groups can be affected.

HISTORY

Ask about the following:

- single joint or multiple?
- antecedent illness or minor trauma?
- fever, malaise, or systemic symptoms?
- medications: warfarin? anti-coagulants?
- family history of arthritis or bleeding disorders?

PHYSICAL EXAM

- swelling truly intra-articular (deep; decreased joint ROM) or more superficial? (in bursa; good ROM)
- signs of sepsis or easy bruising?

LAB AND IMAGING

- CBC; ESR; INR; glucose, creatinine, electrolytes
- Rh factor; uric acid; HLA–B27, etc., as indicated
- X-ray: look for signs of joint involvement or periosteal reaction

DIFFERENTIAL DIAGNOSIS

- common:
  - *osteoarthritic flare-up* (older patient; overuse)
  - *acute gouty attack* (knee, great toe, wrist, or ankle) often associated with stress from recent surgery
  - *hemarthrosis while on warfarin* (minor trauma?)
  - *reactive arthritis* (young people, postviral)
  - *septic arthritis* (de novo in children; in adults: often postorthopaedic surgical intervention, or patients with chronic illness (R/A, CRF, diabetes)

- uncommon, but serious:
  - *new onset inflammatory arthritis* (JRA, ankylosing spondylitis, etc.)
  - *peri-articular tumour* (giant cell tumour, pigmented villonodular synovitis, synovial chondromatosis)
  - *inherited bleeding disorders*

JOINT ASPIRATION

This test can be diagnostic and therapeutic, relieving pain from tense swelling. Sometimes one can clinch the diagnosis immediately once the joint fluid appears in the syringe!

Use sterile technique. Realistically, one can only aspirate the knee, elbow, and subacromial space (potentially shoulder) in the clinic under local anaesthetic. All other joints usually

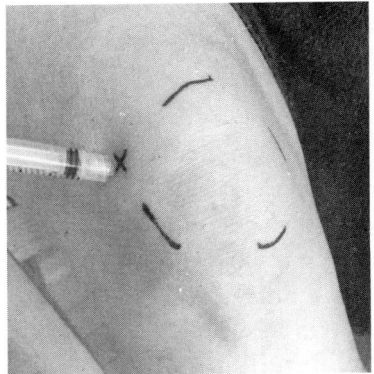

Figure 3.7 Knee aspiration using the superiolateral approach

CHECKLIST FOR JOINT FLUID[6]
- *colour:* bloody; yellow/green (pus); white (gout); turbid beige (inflammatory); clear (reactive or osteoarthritis)
- *viscosity:* reduced in infection and acute inflammation
- *glucose:* reduced in infection
- *cell count:* high in infection; acute inflammation (> 10 WBC/HPF?)
- *crystals:* gout and CPPD
- gram stain and culture

---

need to be aspirated under fluoroscopy, in the X-ray suite, or in the O.R. (especially in children).

The technique for common joint aspiration can be found in Chapter 28.

Most cases of a bloody effusion or frank pus are obvious as soon as the joint fluid enters the syringe. This is good because in the case of septic arthritis, treatment cannot be delayed. Pus is very toxic to joint cartilage, so definitive joint lavage (arthroscopic or open) should be done within 6 hours.

Treatment of most of the other diagnoses is less urgent and usually does not involve joint lavage, but rather treatment of the underlying disorder.

> Pus is very toxic to joint cartilage, so definitive joint lavage (arthroscopic or open) should be done within 6 hours.

Soft Tissue Infections

MSK infections are not limited to joints alone. Infections can affect every layer of the connective tissue from the skin, right down to the bone. *Definitions* of soft tissue infections are important for determining treatment and prognosis:

- local, in skin: furuncle
- local, in skin/fat: carbuncle
- local, in deeper layers: soft tissue abscess
- spreading into skin and fat: cellulitis
- spreading into fascia: fasciitis
- spreading deep into fascia: myonecrosis
- deep, in bone: osteomyelitis

It is crucial to determine the depth and breadth of the infection. The speed of involvement

> It is crucial to determine the depth and breadth of the infection.

and presence of systemic involvement are also very important indicators as to the severity of the infection.

HISTORY
Ask about the following:

- speed of onset; systemic symptoms
- antecedent viral illness (children)
- previous surgery on extremity? metal implant in area
- co-morbidities: diabetes; obesity; IV drug use

PHYSICAL EXAM
Look for the following:

- depth and breadth of involvement
- ecchymosis/petechiae in area (deep, serious infection)
- gas in tissues? (deep infection; not just *Clostridia*)
- regional lymph nodes?
- systemic findings

LAB AND IMAGING

- CBC; ESR: Beware of a very high WBC > 20,000. This denotes a very serious deep infection (fasciitis or myonecrosis).
- electrolytes, creatinine, glucose, INR
- plain X-rays: soft tissue swelling? periosteal reaction? sequestrum in bone?
- ultrasound helpful for fluid-filled soft tissue mass
- bone scan/WBC scan and MRI: helpful in more elective workup of chronic conditions
- infections and soft tissue masses

TREATMENT
There is a real continuum of treatment as the infection goes from localized and superficial to deep and spreading.

- superficial cellulitis: IV antibiotics (gm + *S. aureus*; *S. pyogenes*)
- local abscess: IV antibiotics + drain abscess (+ remove metal implants as required)
- spreading deep infection (fasciitis; necrotizing fasciitis; myonecrosis): resuscitation; IV antibiotics (gram positive and gram negative; *Clostridia*); usually multibacterial; radical debridement (even amputation); hyperbaric oxygen chamber?

Once the infection goes deep into the fascia and starts to spread, these patients become gravely ill. At the end of the spectrum (true necrotizing fasciitis and myonecrosis), the patient can develop septic shock and DIC, with a mortality rate greater than 50% even with treatment. Fortunately, these most aggressive infections are rare and are usually seen in patients with some underlying decrease in their immunity (morbid obesity; diabetes; cancer treatment). Occasionally, a previously healthy patient develops necrotizing fasciitis, for no apparent reason, and these cases can be truly terrifying.

Infection in the Diabetic Foot

Diabetes — and its associated problems — is becoming almost epidemic in Canada as the incidence continues to rise. These infections begin as small areas of skin breakdown that develop into ulcers that do not heal. This is due to a combination of diabetic peripheral neuropathy, possible reduced circulation in the foot, and the impaired immune response often seen in diabetics.

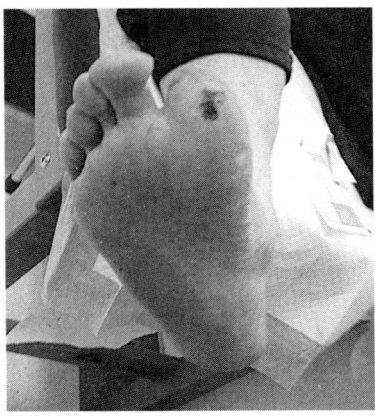

Figure 3.8 Diabetic toe ulcer

Beware of the small toe ulcer over the tip of a toe or a metatarsal head — it can quickly develop into a regional cellulitis that will require IV antibiotics and debridement, and ultimately even a below-knee amputation.

Treatment must be directed toward the foot and the patient's diabetes control in general. Local foot care involves daily cleansing of the ulcer, footwear modifications to get the pressure off the ulcer, and debridement as needed. Regular follow-ups and sometimes home-care visits are required.

If these measures fail, one or more toes may develop dry gangrene and need to be amputated. If this measure fails, below-knee amputation is often required.

Acute Back Pain

Chronic low back pain without neural deficit is exceedingly common in the adult population and should rarely present to the emergency department. A small group of patients, however, present with new or rapidly progressive back and leg pain that can require emergency intervention. Progressive neurologic deficit, from whatever cause, is always a surgical emergency. Progressive loss of bony spinal stability is often associated with progressive neural deficit and must be dealt with simultaneously. This is cauda equina syndrome.

> **Progressive neurologic deficit, from whatever cause, is always a surgical emergency.**

HISTORY

Ask about the following:

- age: 20–40 years = disc disease acute; older than 40 years = degenerative spinal; acute on chronic wide differential diagnosis
- leg pain (sciatica) versus back pain (mechanical) dominant pain
- onset of symptoms; progression? (very important)
- neurologic symptoms: numbness; weakness; bladder and bowel?
- co-morbidities: diabetes; obesity; IV drug abuse; history of cancer?

PHYSICAL EXAM

- systemically ill?
- gait assessment: limp, or cannot walk at all?
- L-spine and hip ROM; better with L-flex = disc/root pain; better with L-extension = facet/mechanical
- detailed neurological exam
- nerve tension tests
- rectal exam (tone and voluntary squeeze on finger)

LAB AND IMAGING

- CBC; ESR; electrolytes; glucose; creatinine
- special tests: blood cultures; alkaline phosphatise; etc.
- plain X-ray: AP; lateral L-spine; AP pelvis; loss of alignment? collapse? asymmetry?
- CT scan: good for bony detail; quick

- bone/WBC scan: useful in infection and tumour workup, needed semi-urgently
- MRI: best for imaging neural elements

An MRI is probably the one best test available when you really need to rule out serious spinal pathology. It can be done on an emergent basis if you call the radiologist. An MRI of spinal infection (pattern of infection versus spinal tumour) is easy to differentiate for the radiologists.

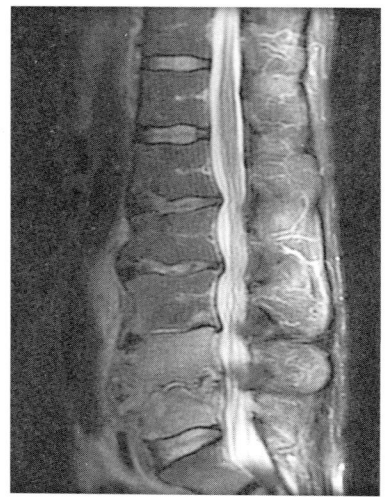

Figure 3.9 MRI of disc and vertebral infection

DIFFERENTIAL DIAGNOSIS

- acute large disc protrusion (lateral > central)
- acute exacerbation of chronic mechanical disc/facet disease (relative spinal stenosis)
- osteoporotic spinal fracture (causes relative spinal stenosis in the elderly spine)
- spinal infection: discitis or vertebral (look for co-morbidity risk factors)
- spinal tumours: usually metastatic > multiple myeloma

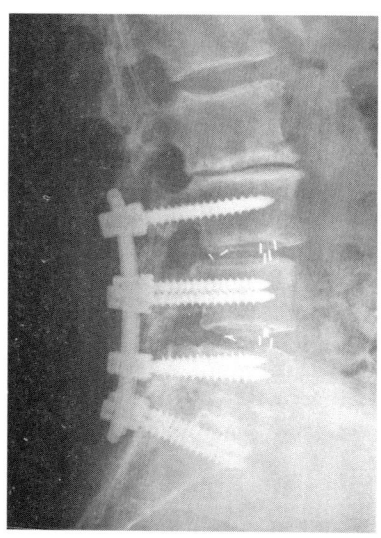

TREATMENT
If the neurological deficit is progressive, the workup and treatment should occur within 12–24 hours. Rapid referral to a tertiary spine centre is indicated.[7]

Figure 3.10 Stabilization of unstable spinal segment

If spinal instability may be present due to a destructive lesion, or fragility fracture, the patient should be kept in bed and log-rolled.

Surgical treatment usually involves decompressing the spinal canal and, often, stabilizing the unstable segments with internal fixation.

Outcomes vary on the underlying cause of cauda equina syndrome. Nerve recovery is quite unpredictable, but the sooner the pressure is relieved on the neural elements the better, particularly if there has been a sudden increase in intracanal pressure.

Child with a Limp

A child with a persistent limp is always of concern since, for them, limps are uncommon in the absence of trauma. There is a spectrum of acuity in the differential diagnosis, so some may present to the office and others to the emergency department. Most problems centre on the hip.

HISTORY
Ask about the following:

- age: very important, as certain disorders only affect one paediatric age group (e.g., Perthes or SCFE)
- painful (most) or painless? (classic = missed DDH)
- rate of onset and trends
- systemic symptoms?
- co-morbidities: obesity? endocrine? DDH as infant?

PHYSICAL EXAM

- well or ill child?
- gait: antalgic or Trendelenburg?
- hip ROM: truly rigid (sepsis); or limited gentle ROM (synovitis)
- chronic contractures of hip? (abduction; external rotation; flexion)
- ROM L-spine and knee
- leg length discrepancy?

LAB AND IMAGING

- CBC; ESR; electrolytes, glucose, creatinine; rheumatoid factor, etc., as indicated
- plain X-ray: AP pelvis; AP; lateral hip; can quickly clinch the diagnosis (DDH; SCFE; Perthes; tumour)
- CT/MRI: reserved for more elective workups, staging

DIFFERENTIAL DIAGNOSIS

- septic arthritis of the hip
- transient synovitis of the hip (viral or post-viral)
- slipped capital femoral epiphysis SCFE of the hip (obese older boys)
- Perthes disease (AVN femoral head) younger boys > girls
- primary bone tumours (Ewings; leukemia; lymphoma; etc.)
- missed DDH (hip dysplasia)

TREATMENT

The major step in diagnosis is to rule out *septic arthritis* of the hip, which is still reasonably common in healthy, usually young children. Pus in the hip can be disastrous to the cartilage and blood supply of the femoral head, so treatment within 12 hours is indicated.

> The major step in diagnosis is to rule out septic arthritis of the hip.

Transient synovitis is more common, and relatively benign, and is the only other diagnosis with similar, though less severe, symptoms and signs as septic arthritis. Usually, the child is less ill than with true septic arthritis and will allow you to move the hip gently. The child's WBC is typically lower as well.

The other major diagnoses are straightforward to rule out on plain X-rays (SCFE; DDH; Perthes; tumour).

If one is reasonably sure the child has transient synovitis of the hip, observation with NSAIDs and re-examination in 12–24 hours is indicated. If one is unsure, the safest thing to do is to take the child to the O.R. and tap the affected hip under flouro guidance (older children could theoretically have this done in the imaging department if they are calm). If the hip aspiration is clear, septic arthritis is ruled out; if it is cloudy or filled with frank pus, the child needs an immediate hip arthrotomy.

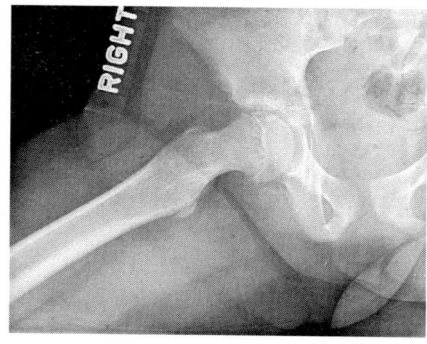

Figure 3.11 Mild SCFE of right hip

The prognosis for septic arthritis is good, but only if the arthrotomy is done early. If the diagnosis is missed, the child is headed for growth problems of the hip/femur and early hip arthritis.

In conclusion, these nine urgent orthopaedic conditions/scenarios are very important, and one needs an approach to deal with each of these in community practice. They are either common, or serious, and should be familiar to every family doctor.

REFERENCES

1. Mohammad A, Branicki F, Abu-Zidan FM. Educational and clinical impact of Advanced Trauma Life Support (ATLS) courses: a systematic review. *World J Surg.* 2014;38(2):322–9.

2. Behrman SW, Fabian TC, Kudsk KA, et al. Improved outcome with femur fractures: early vs. delayed fixation. *J Trauma.* 1990;30(7):792–8, discussion 797–8. http://dx.doi.org/10.1097/00005373-199007000-00005. Medline:2380996

3. Gustilo RB, Merkow RL, Templeman D. The management of open fractures. *J Bone Joint Surg Am.* 1990;72(2):299–304. Medline:2406275

4. Pape HC, Tornetta III P, Tarkin I, et al. Timing of fracture fixation in multitrauma patients: the role of early total care and damage control surgery. *J Am Acad Orthop Surg.* 2009;17(9):541–9. Medline:19726738

5. Klippel JH, editor. Joint fluid analysis. *Primer on the Rheumatic Diseases.* 13th ed. Springer; 2008. p. 23–6. http://dx.doi.org/10.1007/978-0-387-68566-3.

6. Shadgan B, Menon M, Sanders D, et al. Current thinking about acute compartment syndrome of the lower extremity. *Can J Surg.* 2010;53(5):329–34. Medline:20858378

7. Gleave JRW, Macfarlane R. Cauda equina syndrome: what is the relationship between timing of surgery and outcome? *Br J Neurosurg.* 2002;16(4):325–8. http://dx.doi.org/10.1080/0268869021000032887. Medline:12389883

PART TWO

ORTHOPAEDIC TRAUMA IN ADULTS

4

General Principles of Orthopaedic Trauma

Describing a plain X-ray is a critical skill for primary-care physicians and is mandatory in fractures and dislocations. (Please see Chapter 2 for a detailed discussion of X-rays.) In brief, X-rays should be in two planes 90 degrees to each other and include the joints above and below the injury. Description includes the following:

- age of patient
- open or closed injury
- displaced or nondisplaced
- LARA

> Describing a plain X-ray is a critical skill for primary-care physicians.

- Location: which bone? where in bone? intra-articular?
- Apposition of fracture fragments
- Rotation (long bones)
- Angulation: distal relative to proximal fragment; where is apex of deformity?

Please see Chapter 3 for a timetable of fracture treatment; a detailed discussion of multiple trauma and orthopaedics; open fractures and their treatment in the emergency department; closed fractures and dislocations in the emergency department (relative frequency and primary-care treatment); and compartment syndrome/swollen limbs.

General Principles of Adult Fractures

The two most important features of the orthopaedic history are (1) the age of the patient, which predicts the fracture pattern expected and the weak link, and (2) the amount of energy involved — high or low — in producing the injury. These concepts were introduced in Chapter 1 but are worth repeating.

Age and Weak Link

Although some injuries occur over various age groups, at every stage of life, around every joint, usually one part of the bone/joint complex is the weakest. With a force applied, the failure will predictably occur at this weak link.

Examples:

- *young children:* greenstick fractures (due to flexible long bones)
- *teenagers:* growth plate injuries (usually Salter II)
- *young adults:* ligament injuries (knee) and dislocations; scaphoid fractures (due to strong bones; fused growth plates)
- *elderly:* hip and metaphyseal fractures; fragility fractures; cuff tears (due to osteoporosis or thinning of the soft tissues)

Any fracture pattern is possible at any age with enough force, but in general, one can predict where the weak spot will be and what fracture pattern will be present on X-ray based on the age of the patient.

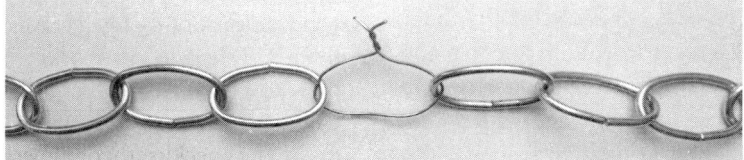

Figure 4.1 Age predicts where the weak link lies.

Energy Level

The energy level of the injury predicts the amount of bone and soft tissue damage initially and is predictive of the ease of repair, time to healing, and complication rate. All become more problematic as the amount of energy increases. Post-traumatic problems presenting even years afterward can often be traced back to a high-energy injury. Most orthopaedic fracture classification systems consider this factor, as they are predictive of outcome:[1]

- *low energy:* nondisplaced or minimal fragmentation
- *medium energy:* displaced, often intra-articular
- *high energy:* widely displaced; comminuted fractures (often with significant soft tissue injury or open wounds)

Most systems use A, B, C or 1, 2, 3 to denote the increasing energy levels involved and the increasing complexity of the fracture. Open fractures are

> Most orthopaedic fracture classification systems are based on the energy level needed to produce the injury.

graded in a similar fashion related to the size of the open wound, again dependent on the amount of energy involved in producing the injury.[2]

Predicting Outcome in Fracture Care

Several general indicators predict outcome in fracture care. First, by definition, what is a successful fracture outcome? Success for fracture recovery means not only a healed fracture, but also a return to pre-injury levels of activities of daily living (ADL), work, sports, and hobbies. Radiographic fracture healing is only part of the equation for success, and patient expectations vary widely depending on age, occupation, and interests.

Most fractures take about 3 months to heal; this time may decrease in younger people and simple fracture patterns and increase with age and other

> Success = a healed fracture *and* a return to pre-injury levels of activities of daily living, work, sports, and hobbies.

complicating factors, such as those shown in the checklist that follows.

CHECKLIST OF FACTORS THAT PREDICT FRACTURE CARE OUTCOME

Fracture specific

- *amount of energy involved in the injury:* low energy (do well); high energy (predict problems early on with fixation and late with complications)
- *age and fracture pattern:* age will predict where the weak link is; certain fracture patterns are more difficult to fix, particularly if they are intra-articular or comminuted
- *quality of the bone:* poor (osteoporotic) bone, does not hold fixation well, collapses during healing, and heals more slowly

- *single extremity or multiple limb injury:* at least double the time to recovery after more than one extremity is injured (3 months to more than 6 months); multiple trauma patients take at least 1 year to recover

Patient specific

- *age:* apart from predicting the fracture pattern to expect; age does affect the speed of bone healing and recovery in a more or less linear pattern
- *co-morbidities:* all increase the risk of complications and prolong the recovery phase: obesity; diabetes; chronic renal failure; rheumatoid arthritis; heart and lung disease; steroid use; dementia
- *social factors:* level of independence before the injury (in the elderly); cigarette smoking (delays bone healing; wound healing); alcohol or substance abuse (compliance and truth issues)
- *work history:* WCB injuries take longer to return successfully to work (up to 50% longer[3]); in my experience, self-employed farmers and ranchers successfully return to work the quickest

Complications

Complications can be early or late, local or systemic, and all can lead to a poor outcome.

CHECKLIST OF COMMON FRACTURE COMPLICATIONS

Early local

- *neurovascular injury/compromise* (usually at the time of the original injury)*:* vessels can be repaired; nerves are more unpredictable
- *wound breakdown/infection:* more common in high-energy injuries; smokers; diabetics; obesity
- *loss of initial reduction or fixation:* poor bone; bad fracture pattern

Early systemic

- *DVT → PTE:* proximal lower limb; predictable risk factors
- *sepsis* (wound; urine; chest)*: →* ARDS (multiple trauma)
- *cardiac events:* myocardial infarct (MI), arrhythmias post-operative

Late local (weeks → months)

- *joint stiffness:* probably the most common problem with all adult fractures
- *malunion:* fracture has healed, but position suboptimal
- *delayed-union:* fracture is slow to heal, but still progressing (less than 6 months)
- *nonunion:* all signs of fracture healing have stopped (usually more than 6 months)
- *post-traumatic arthritis:* high-energy intra-articular fractures

- *avascular necrosis (AVN):* hip; scaphoid; talus; humeral head
- *RSDS:* upper limb injuries

Late systemic (months → years)

- *loss of work/occupation:* Even if the fracture heals, the outcome will be compromised if the patient is unable to do his or her pre-injury job, particularly in occupations that require heavy lifting or repetitive use of the upper extremity.

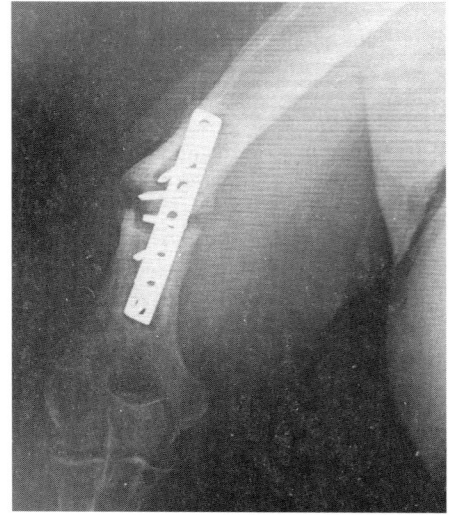

Figure 4.2 Late nonunion of humerus fracture despite plating

- *loss of independence:* Many elderly patients are just managing to cope at home independently before the fracture. A fracture will tip them over the threshold so they may not be able to live independently for 3–6 months afterward; often, this is a permanent change in living arrangement.

- *mobility:* There is a rule of thumb that elderly patients go *down* one level of ambulation (for at least 3–6 months) after a fracture (i.e., no walking aide → cane; cane → walker; walker → wheelchair).

> Elderly patients generally go *down* one level of ambulation function after a significant fracture.

General Indications for Open Reduction/Fixation

A default list of general indications is helpful before specific fractures by anatomic region are discussed in the following chapters. Regardless of the anatomic site of the fracture, these indications usually apply:[4]

- *open fractures:* Any open fracture, regardless of the size of the wound, will need debridement; some sort of open reduction and internal fixation usually follows.

- *displaced intra-articular fractures* (2 mm or greater): Because of the risk of post-traumatic stiffness and arthritis, these fractures should be fixed so the joint is as anatomic as possible.

- *fractures in poly-trauma:* Even if the fracture itself is treated conservatively, we tend to be more aggressive with getting these patients upright and out of bed quickly to minimize chest, DVT, and sepsis; upper-extremity slings and casts also poorly tolerated with chest and belly injuries.

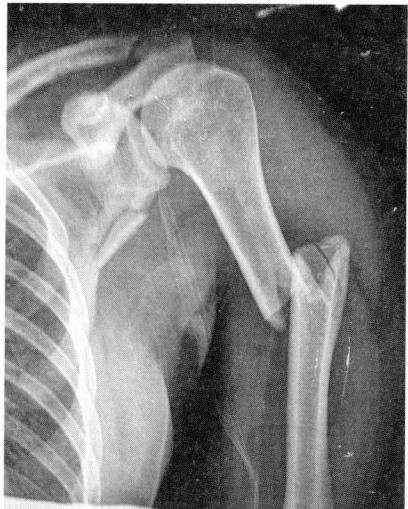

Figure 4.3 X-ray demonstrating floating limb: fractured left scapula and left humeral shaft

- *floating limb:* If patients have fractures on both sides of a joint (e.g., clavicle and humerus fracture), fix one or both for mobility and ADL.

- *unstable fracture patterns:* The following fracture patterns in adults either displace or heal unacceptably slowly in a splint or cast:
  · displaced both bones of forearm
  · Holstein's (distal third) shaft fracture of humerus
  · extra-articular wrist fractures; with comminution, poor bone
  · spinal fractures with 2 or 3 columns affected
  · displaced hip fractures
  · displaced tibial and femoral shaft fractures

The Big Four

In community orthopaedic practice, four areas are most commonly injured, providing the majority of orthopaedic traumas:

1. hip fractures
2. ankle fractures/injuries
3. wrist fractures/injuries
4. knee injuries (both soft tissue and bone)

These four areas are covered in the next four chapters, followed by other anatomic areas seen less frequently.

REFERENCES

1. Bucholz RW, Heckman JD, Tornetta III P. editors *Rockwood and Green's fractures in adults*; 7th ed. 2009 p. 41; Lippincott.
2. Gustilo RB, Merkow RL, Templeman D. The management of open fractures. *J Bone Joint Surg Am.* 1990;72(2):299–304. Medline:2406275
3. Seland K, Cherry N, Beach J. A study of factors influencing return to work after wrist or ankle fractures. *Am J Ind Med.* 2006;49(3):197–203. http://dx.doi.org/10.1002/ajim.20258. Medline:16421918
4. Bucholz RW, Heckman JD, Tornetta III P. editors *Rockwood and Green's fractures in adults*; 7th ed. 2009; p. 913; Lippincott.

5

Hip

Demographics

Hip fractures are extremely common and, because of the advancing age of the population, are increasing in frequency. The average age of patients with hip fractures is also increasing, for various reasons.[1] At a busy hospital, hip fractures are seen on a daily basis, occurring year-round, regardless of weather conditions. You may hear someone say, "The weather is bad. You'll see lots of broken hips today!" But this is not true. Broken hips occur most frequently in elderly people who generally stay indoors when the weather is treacherous.

Typically, an elderly patient, whose balance is borderline to begin with, trips over a small step or irregularity in the flooring and falls to the ground. The patient is often trapped in that spot for hours before help arrives, becoming quite dehydrated by the time he or she reaches the hospital.

> Hip fractures are, generally, an indoor, low-energy injury.

The corollary of these generalizations is that if you do see a hip fracture in a younger patient, it is unusual and you should beware. It is a high-energy injury, is more difficult to treat, and has a different personality than the typical hip fracture in the elderly.

Mechanism of Injury

Mechanism of injury is an important concept, as it predicts the type of fracture that will occur; it is not stressed enough in standard texts.

NO PRE-EXISTING HIP-JOINT OSTEOARTHRITIS

These patients have good range of motion in their hip joints, so when they lose their balance and fall at low speed, they flex and twist as they fall. The weak spot in elderly bone is the femoral neck, so the twisting motion actually fractures the femoral neck *before* they hit the ground.

These patients have intracapsular femoral neck fractures on X-ray. In hemi-arthroplasty surgery, the hip joint cartilage is usually pristine.

PRE-EXISTING HIP-JOINT OSTEOARTHRITIS

These patients have arthritic hips and are stiff; when they lose their balance they cannot flex, so they fall over "like a ton of bricks" directly onto the lateral side of their hip. The hip does not break until it hits the ground. These patients sustain extracapsular, intertrochanteric, or more distal fractures. Sometimes, they can be quite comminuted and widely displaced, even after a ground-level fall.

Classification

Hip fracture classification is important because it predicts prognosis for healing and, therefore, treatment. The ability of the fracture to heal in the hip is largely based on blood supply. The hip is one of the unique areas of the body with a *retrograde blood supply*, so the femoral head is at risk of avascular necrosis and/or nonunion if the blood supply is disrupted. Therefore, we can classify hip fractures according to blood supply and amount of displacement, and then subclassify them anatomically.

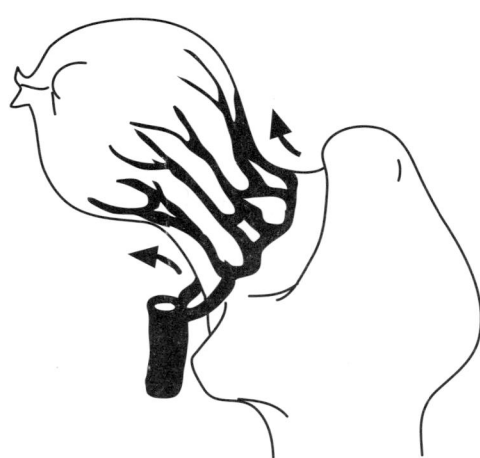

Figure 5.1 Diagram of femoral head blood supply: Ninety percent is retrograde.

INTRACAPSULAR FRACTURES (NONDISPLACED/IMPACTED OR DISPLACED)

- subcapital femoral neck (most common)
- transcervical femoral neck

The femoral head circulation is disrupted in these fractures if the fracture is displaced. AVN and nonunion are complications. There is usually no pre-existing arthritis of the hip joint.

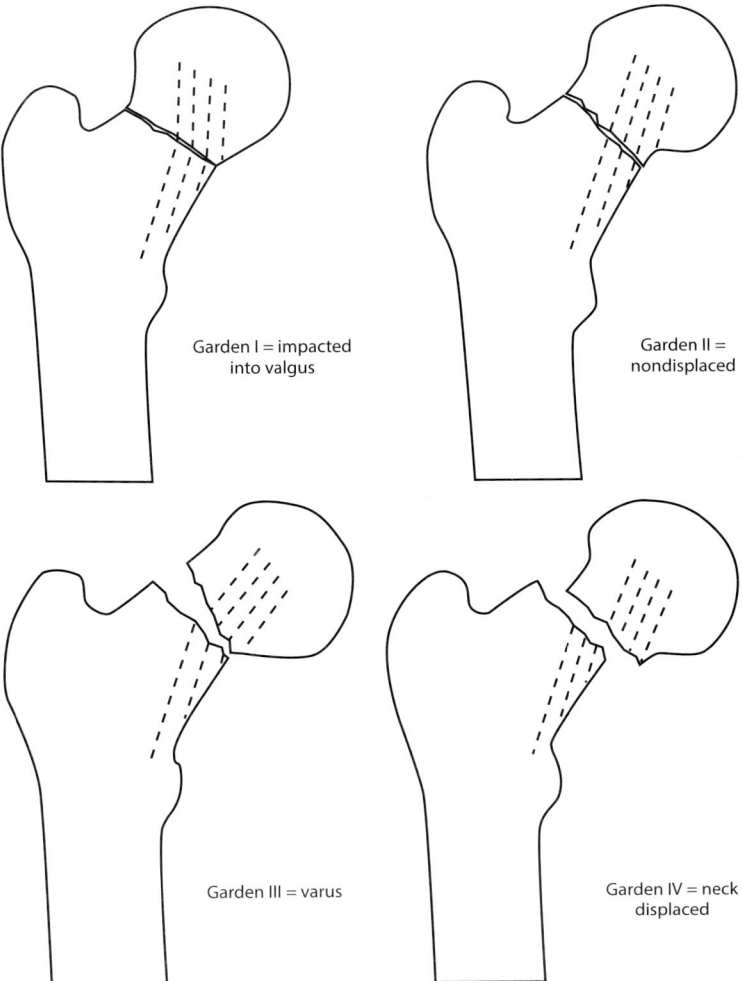

Garden I = impacted into valgus

Garden II = nondisplaced

Garden III = varus

Garden IV = neck displaced

Figure 5.2 The Garden classification system is used with femoral neck fractures.

EXTRACAPSULAR FRACTURES (NONDISPLACED OR DISPLACED)

- *intertrochanteric* (most common site, most displaced)
- *subtrochanteric* (look for horrendous clinical varus deformity; often very frail, very elderly patients)
- *low basicervical* (many nondisplaced or minimally displaced); right at junction of neck and trochanteric line; act and treated like tricky intertrochanteric fractures (more difficult to reduce and fix)

All these fractures will heal and all have an excellent blood supply — in fact, bleeding can be a problem in these patients. Malunion, not nonunion, is the problem here, often worsening a pre-existing arthritic hip, which predisposes patients to this mechanism of injury. Deforming muscle forces around the hip are strong, so rigid, large implants are required.

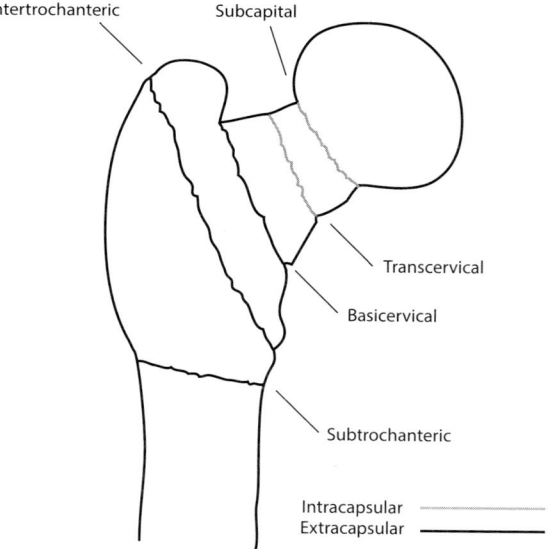

Figure 5.3 Drawing demonstrating anatomic sites of hip fractures

Emergency Treatment

Treatment of all hip fractures is *primarily supportive*. These patients are elderly and often frail, and they are frequently dehydrated from lying at home with their hip fracture before help arrived.

- Start IV fluids.
- Restart home meds missed (except anticoagulants).
- Watch for areas of skin breakdown.
- Start antibiotics if chest, urine, or skin at risk.
- Check status of INR, hemoglobin, electrolytes, creatinine.
- Medical consult is often prudent.

Operative treatment ideally should occur within 48 hours of the injury, so these patients do not have to be kept fasting initially.

Operative Treatment

Intracapsular Fractures

NONDISPLACED/IMPACTED

Nondisplaced/Impacted intracapsular hip fractures are usually Type A (subcapital location) or mild valgus Garden I and II types. Occasionally, these impacted fractures can just be monitored with serial X-rays if the patient has minimal pain and moves the hip well. More commonly, the hip is too painful to move or walk on. Operative treatment includes in-situ screw fixation, protected weight bearing for 3 months, and monitoring for AVN.

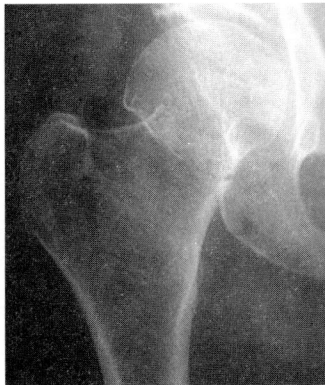

Figure 5.4 Impacted (valgus) subcapital hip fracture

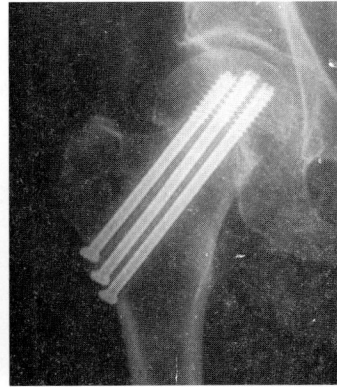

Figure 5.5 In-situ screw fixation for impacted subcapital hip fracture

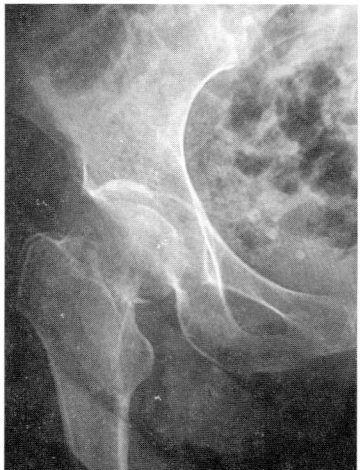

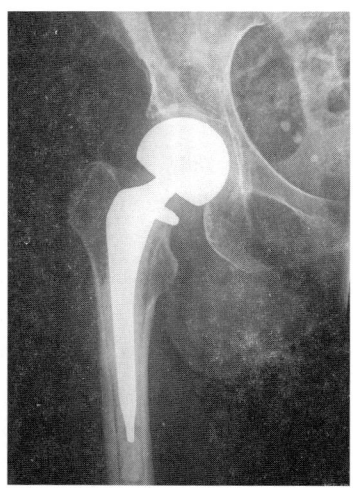

Figure 5.6 Displaced transcervical hip fracture (Note varus position.)

Figure 5.7 Hemi-arthroplasty for displaced intracapsular hip fracture in the elderly

DISPLACED

Displaced intracapsular hip fractures feature the head in varus with little or no contact with distal fragment on the lateral view. By definition, the blood supply has been disrupted and the femoral is at risk of AVN and nonunion. In the elderly, this is not a problem, and we routinely perform a hemi-arthroplasty. These patients do very well and can fully weight bear immediately. In younger, active patients (which is, fortunately, relatively rare), arthroplasty is not ideal. This situation may become a relative emergency and the fracture reduction and screw fixation must be done within 12–24 hours. This is the only real indication for emergency hip surgery.

Extracapsular Fractures

DISPLACED, INTERTROCHANTERIC

Displaced, intertrochanteric hip fractures are straightforward and do well. Occasionally, they are more comminuted, and 3- and 4-part fractures are more difficult to reduce and hold and they often shorten with healing. Fixation methods include DHS (dynamic hip screw) or a short intramedullary device (Gamma or TFN).

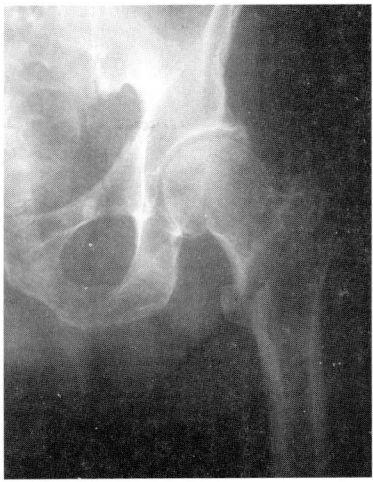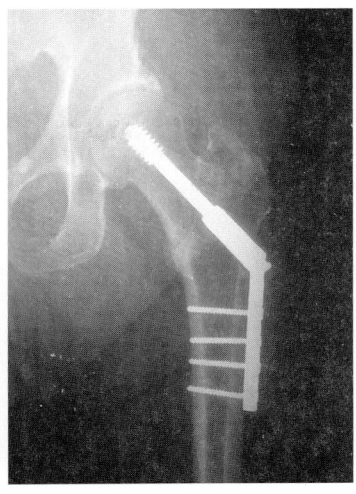

Figure 5.8 Displaced intertrochanteric left hip fracture

Figure 5.9 Fixation with DHS implant (left intertrochanteric hip fracture)

DISPLACED, SUBTROCHANTERIC

Displaced, subtrochanteric hip fractures are higher-energy injuries. In frailer patients, blood loss can be significant, and the fracture cannot be held with a standard DHS implant. Instead, a large intramedullary device is needed to counter the varus deforming forces.

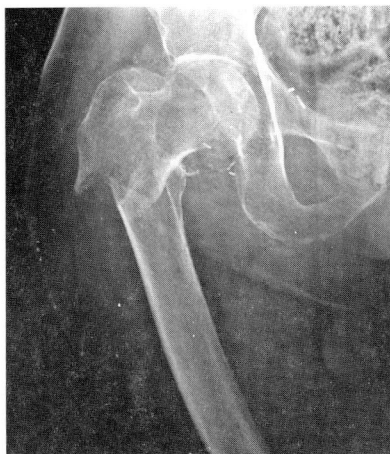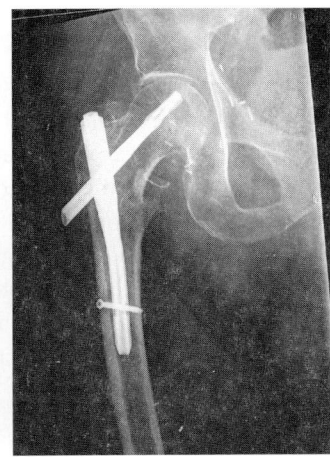

Figure 5.10 Subtrochanteric fracture (collapses into varus) (Note typical marked deformity.)

Figure 5.11 Fixation with intramedullary device

DISPLACED, LOW BASICERVICAL

Displaced, low basicervical hip fractures are a variant of intertrochanteric fractures, but less common, and more difficult to reduce and fix in the O.R. DHS is a good implant for this fracture.

Complications

Hip fractures are common and the elderly have many co-morbidities, so one should expect some postoperative complications. Normal hip fractures take 3–6 months to heal, and *patients will not return to their full level of functioning for 6–12 months*,

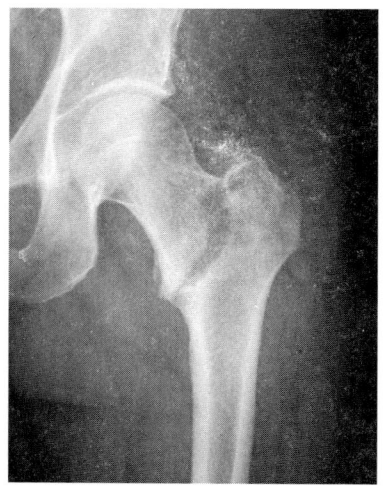

Figure 5.12 Low basilar displaced hip fracture

even without major complications. The biggest complication, ultimately, is death, and the mortality rate in hip fracture care is significant.

The mortality rate *after surgically treated* hip fractures is still quite high, not necessarily in the immediate postoperative period (5–10%), but can approach 25% if patients are followed for the whole year after surgery.[2] Death generally results from medical complications: DVT/PTE, heart and lung disease, worsening of CRF, etc. The biggest predictors of mortality are the age of the patient (> 80 years), the number of co-morbidities, and the presence of significant dementia.[3]

We tend to treat almost all patients with hip fractures surgically, even if they have significant dementia — to get them out of bed and mobile. Early mortality *without surgery* is very high

> **Almost all hip fractures are treated surgically in order to get patients mobile.**

(more than 50% within the first month) and the hip fracture itself is so painful that it usually requires bedrest, which is bad for elderly people. Death usually comes in the form of sepsis (lung, urine, or skin breakdown) or multisystem failure.

CHECKLIST OF HIP FRACTURE COMPLICATIONS

Early local

- *wound problems:* bleeding; infection; drainage
- *DVT:* prophylaxis should be routine unless contraindications; rates > 50% without prophylaxis; rates still 20–40% with prophylaxis, but fewer PTE[4]
- *early loss of fixation:* especially subtrochanteric fractures

Early systemic

- *confusion postoperative:* very common, very distressing to families; cause usually multifactoral; resolves in days with supportive care; R/O metabolic cause first
- *cardiac:* arrhythmias (usually rapid atrial fibrillation) and postoperative myocardial infarction
- *hypoxia:* PTE; CHF; pneumonia
- *renal failure:* acute or chronic
- *anemia:* transfusions are common; particularly with subtrochanteric and comminuted intertrochanteric fractures

Late local

- *delayed or nonunions:* in impacted intracapsular fractures treated with screws < 10% cases
- *joint chondrolysis:* after hemi-arthroplasty (< 5%); increased pain and decreased joint space over time

Late systemic

- *loss of independence:* permanent change in living arrangements
- *ambulation goes down one level* (for at least 3–6 months): no walking aide → cane; cane → walker; walker → wheelchair
- *increased mortality rate:* for up to 1 year

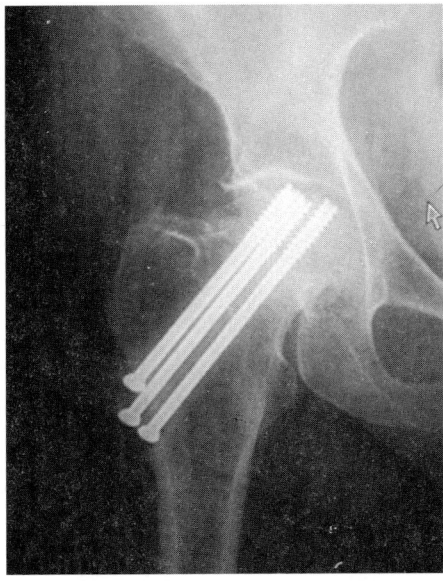

Figure 5.13 AVN and joint chondrolysis after femoral neck fixation

REFERENCES

1. Papadimitropoulos EA, Coyte PC, Josse RG, et al. Current and projected rates of hip fracture in Canada. *CMAJ*. 1997;157(10):1357–63. Medline:9371065

2. Weller I, Wai EK, Jaglal S, et al. The effect of hospital type and surgical delay on mortality after surgery for hip fracture. *J Bone Joint Surg Br*. 2005;87-B(3):361–6. http://dx.doi.org/10.1302/0301-620X.87B3.15300. Medline:15773647

3. Richmond J, Aharonoff GB, Zuckerman JD, et al. Mortality risk after hip fracture. *J Orthop Trauma*. 2003;17(1):53–6. http://dx.doi.org/10.1097/00005131-200301000-00008. Medline:12499968

4. Beaupre LA, Jones CA, Saunders LD, et al. Best practices for elderly hip fracture patients. A systematic overview of the evidence. *J Gen Intern Med*. 2005;20(11):1019–25. http://dx.doi.org/10.1111/j.1525-1497.2005.00219.x. Medline:16307627

6

Ankle

Ankle injuries are exceedingly common for all age groups, especially when the weather turns inclement and it is slippery outdoors. Broadly speaking, there are two major categories of ankle injuries: low-energy slips and high-energy impaction/shearing injuries (Pilon fractures).

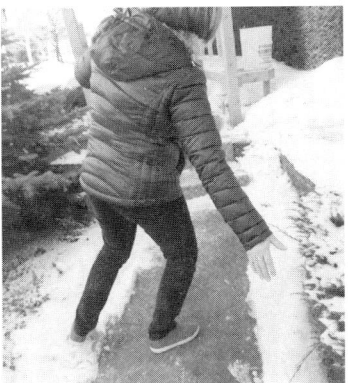

Figure 6.1 Typical low-energy ankle fracture mechanism

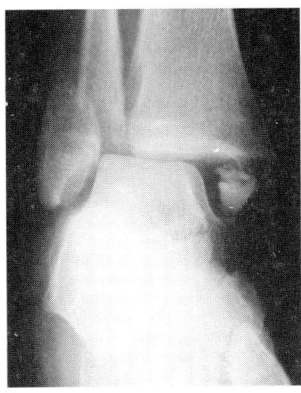

Figure 6.2 Low-energy external rotation valgus injury (80% of ankle fractures)

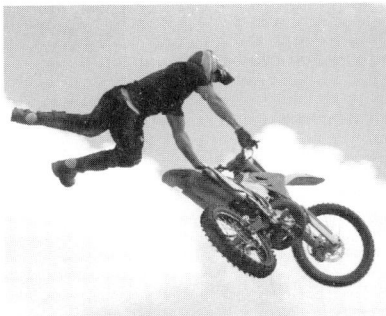

Figure 6.3 High-energy ankle/Pilon fracture scenario

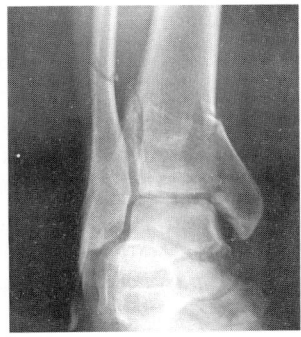

Figure 6.4 High-energy, Pilon-type ankle fracture

Classification of Ankle Fractures

The major decision regarding treatment of ankle fractures is determining which fracture patterns are stable in a cast and which require surgical fixation. Look for a shift in the ankle mortise and two or more malleoli fractured to predict instability.

Ankle fracture classifications should include the following:

1. number of malleoli fractured

   (medial, lateral, posterior); two or more = unstable

2. symmetry of ankle mortise

   (any shift = unstable)

3. location of fibular fracture

   (below, at level of, or above joint line; above = unstable)

The Weber system is widely taught but can be confusing for learners.

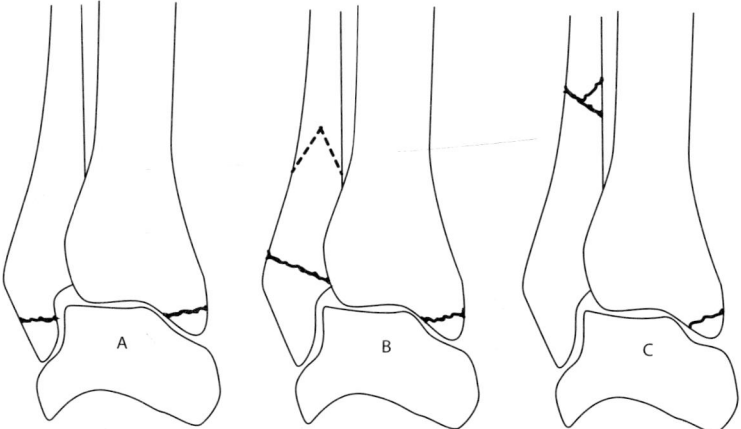

Figure 6.5 Weber (A/O) classification system: based on level of fibular fracture

As an alternative to the Weber system, simply count the number of malleoli involved (or ligament equivalents) and name it accordingly — single malleoli, bimalleolar, trimalleolar — plus or minus a subluxation/dislocation; then comment on whether the ankle mortise is perfect or asymmetrical.

If the ankle is subluxed or dislocated, the foot typically goes laterally and posteriorly (in most low- to medium-energy typical ankle fractures).

If the ankle mortise is shifted and you do not see a malleolar frac-

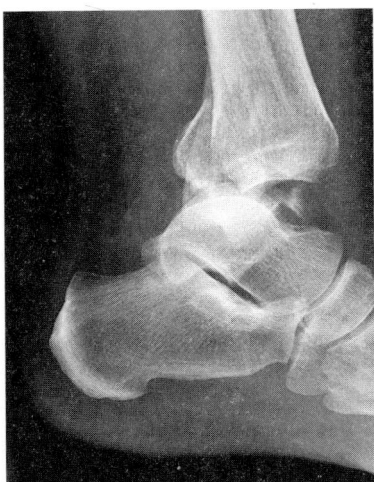 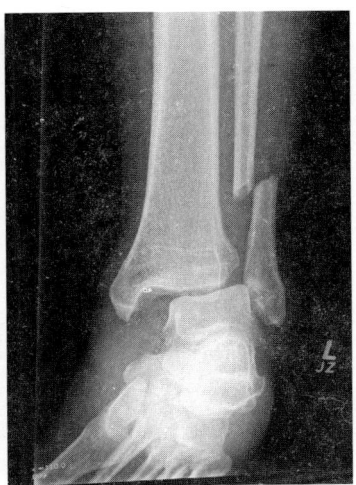

Figure 6.6 Posterior ankle fracture/
dislocation

Figure 6.7 Note the asymmetrical,
widened medially, ankle mortise. (The
deltoid ligament has ruptured and the
fibular fracture is high.) = bimalleolar
fracture equivalent (Weber C)

ture, look for a high fibular fracture and a medial (deltoid) ligament
injury.

High-energy ankle fractures are unstable by definition. The fracture classification systems here look more at the degree of damage
to the joint surface and the degree of reconstructive difficulty that
results. The Pilon fracture classification system, for example, includes
the following:

A = extra-articular (metaphyseal)

B = intra-articular (large chunks)

C = extra- and intra-articular, add 1, 2, or 3 depending on degree
of comminution

Emergency Room Treatment

Regardless of the type of ankle fracture, if there is a deformity, you
must realign and splint the extremity in order to take the pressure off
the soft tissues and improve circulation to the foot. Some of these frac-
ture/dislocations are really quite markedly crooked — the good news
is that they are so unstable, they are easy to reduce as well.

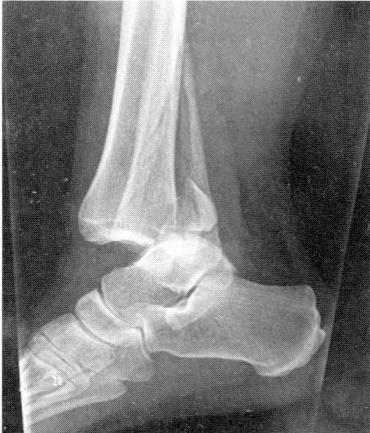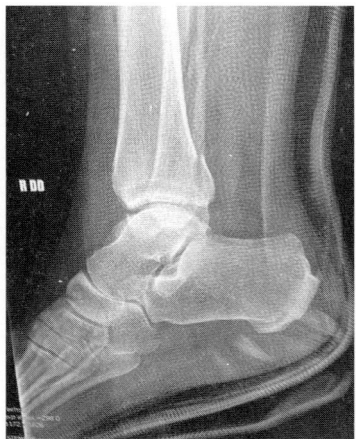

Figure 6.8 Posterior ankle fracture/dislocation before and after realignment

Operative Treatment

Once realigned, most ankle fractures should be fixed within a few days. Pilon fractures often need to be realigned, externally fixated, and then brought back to the O.R. 10–14 days later when the soft tissues are healthier.

Principles of ankle open reduction internal fixation (ORIF):

- fibula out to length
- ankle joint surface congruent
- mortise reduced and stable (Use diastasis screw if necessary.)

Healing Times

Most ankle fractures take 3 months to heal:

- 1 month crutches (non-weight bearing)
- 1 month walking cast or air boot
- 1 month for physiotherapy

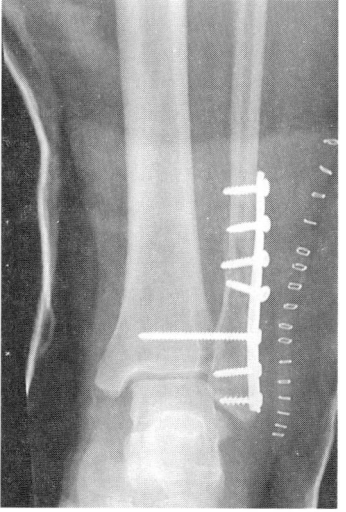

Figure 6.9 The long screw is a diastasis screw (bimalleolar fracture equivalent; torn deltoid ligament).

- Healing times are longer in the following cases:
  - diabetics; peripheral vascular disease; obese patients
  - higher-energy injuries (Pilon fractures take 6–12 months to heal.)

Complications

Obesity, vascular disease, and Pilon fractures may all pose complications for ankle recovery. Diabetics have longer healing times and higher complication rates around the foot and ankle for several reasons:

- *peripheral neuropathy:* feel little pain after surgery → walk on ankle too early → fixation pulls out → loss of fixation → wound breaks down
- *small vessel disease:* delayed wound and fracture healing
- *immune compromise:* increase in infection; poor wound healing

These factors are obviously related to the severity of the diabetes and its complications, including number of years on insulin and the overall compliance of the patient.

CHECKLIST OF ANKLE FRACTURE COMPLICATIONS

Early
- wound breakdown; infection

Late
- ankle stiffness (most common problem)
- persistent swelling (normal to last 6 months)
- loss of fixation; deep infection (diabetics, in particular)
- chondrolysis; post-traumatic osteoarthritis (higher-energy injuries with crush or shear component)

Ankle Sprains

Sprained ankles are very common injuries seen in primary care, but they seldom require orthopaedic surgical intervention. Typically, they occur in teenagers and younger adults with strong bones and loose joints and ligaments, often with a history of chronic weak ankles. Risk factors include generalized ligamentous laxity and jumping/twisting sports such as basketball and soccer.

The typical mechanism of injury is an inversion/varus injury — just the opposite of the typical external rotation valgus-type ankle fracture. The lateral ligament complex (calcaneal talo fibular ligament) partially or fully tears. Avulsion fractures from the tip of the fibula are possible but usually very small and distal.

Treatment acutely is non-operative but should be stringent. If the lateral ligaments are allowed to heal in a lax position, chronic instability may result. (See Chapter 27 for discussion of chronic ankle rollers.) Most recommend neutral ankle splinting/crutches/non-weight bearing until the swelling has decreased (2 weeks) and then convert to a walking cast or air boot for the subsequent 4 weeks. The ankle can dorsi- and plantarflex, but it should not be moved into varus (medially) for 6 weeks until physiotherapy starts. Risky sports should be avoided for 3 months.

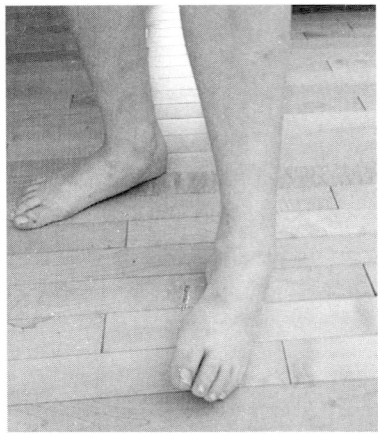

Figure 6.10 Typical mechanism for common ankle sprain (Note opposite mechanism to common valgus low-energy ankle fractures.)

Achilles Tendon Injuries

In the emergency department, these are common injuries with classic histories. Typically, patients are in the 30- to 50-year age group and participating in an intense running/jumping/lunging sport, usually not on a regular basis. They describe a sudden sharp pain in their lower calf as if "someone kicked me from behind," but no one is usually nearby. They have difficulty walking and usually sit out the rest of the game.

Most patients present within 24–48 hours of the injury with calf swelling, weakness in toe

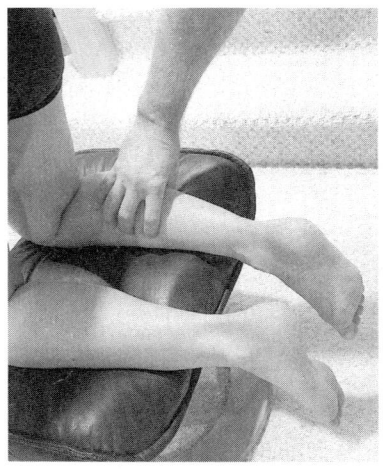

Figure 6.11 Thompson test is positive if no passive plantar flexion of foot on affected side.

push-off, and a limp. Full-thickness tears show a palpable gap in the tendon just proximal to the insertion into the calcaneus. Active plantarflexion will be intact [from the other plantarflexors that cross the ankle (FHL; FDL)], but active heel raises are impossible.

Full-thickness tears are quite easy to diagnose; partial-thickness tears (or tears more proximal in the muscle than its insertion) can be more difficult to detect. The passive calf squeeze test (Thompson test) is quite reliable. Have the patient prone (or kneel on a chair); then gently squeeze the normal and then the abnormal calf. If the Achilles tendon is intact, the foot should passively plantarflex. If it is a complete tear, the foot remains in the neutral position (a positive Thompson test). An ultrasound can be done quickly to confirm the level of the tear and whether it is partial or full thickness.

Treatment

PARTIAL-THICKNESS TEARS

- nonoperative
- below-knee splint/crutches → gradual increase in weight bearing with air boot → physiotherapy

FULL-THICKNESS TEARS

- usually early operative repair
- if patient healthy, no significant co-morbidities
- end-to-end suture repair → non-weight bearing
- below-knee splint/crutches → air boot at 3–4 weeks → physiotherapy

These injuries still take 3 months to heal. Often, patients never fully regain the strength and elasticity of the calf muscles for running sports.

In some regions of the world, even full-thickness tears are treated without surgery, with careful splinting and casting, gradually getting the foot out of plantarflexion. The results are not much different from the operative group after 2 years.[1] Patient compliance with serial casting is the key factor with this method of treatment.

REFERENCE

1. Kocher MS, Bishop J, Marshall R, et al. Operative versus nonoperative management of acute Achilles tendon rupture: expected-value decision analysis. *Am J Sports Med.* 2002;30(6):783–90. Medline:12435641

7

Wrist

Wrist injuries are very common in all age groups. They are seen commonly when the weather makes sidewalks slippery (along with broken ankles) in older adults, in sports-related accidents in young people, and in many falls from heights and motor vehicle accidents. Clinically, they often present with a "dinner fork deformity."

We can make some broad generalizations regarding wrist injuries over the lifespan because the weak link around the wrist changes with age. Therefore, with a fall on the outstretched hand/wrist, we see different injury patterns:

- *under 15–17 years* = Salter II distal radius fractures
- *18–25 years* (particularly males) = scaphoid fractures
- *25–45 years* = ligament tears (strains); metaphyseal fractures (more complex nature; higher energy needed to break these stronger bones)
- *45 years* = metaphyseal fractures (Colles' type and variants)

Overall, most wrist fractures are low energy and do well with closed reduction and casting (often with the addition of percutaneous pins). However, there are certain **features that predict instability of wrist fractures** and may point to future complications:

- high-energy mechanism of injury:
  - · marked initial displacement of fragments

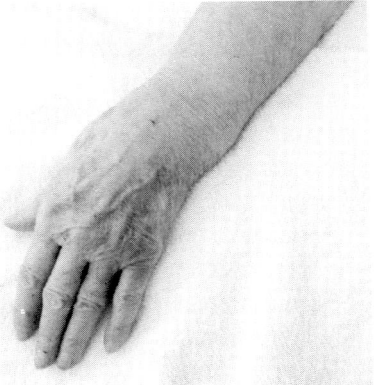

Figure 7.1 Typical appearance of a Colles' wrist fracture

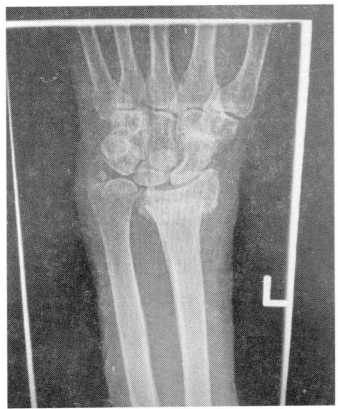

Figure 7.2 Low-energy, Colles' type extra-articular wrist fracture

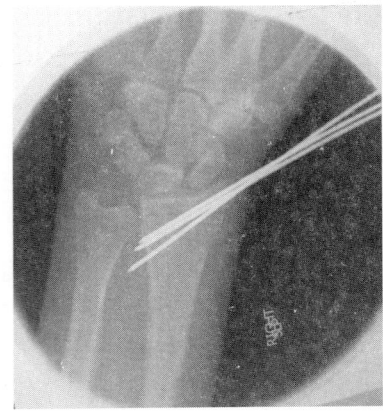

Figure 7.3 Percutaneous pinning of low-energy extra-articular wrist fracture

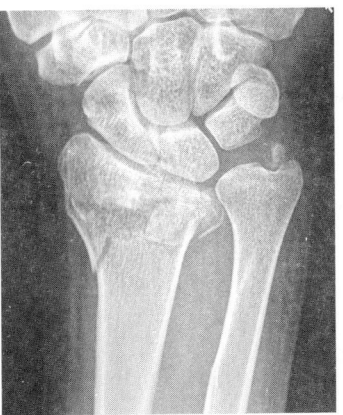

Figure 7.4 Higher-energy, 3-part intra-articular wrist fracture

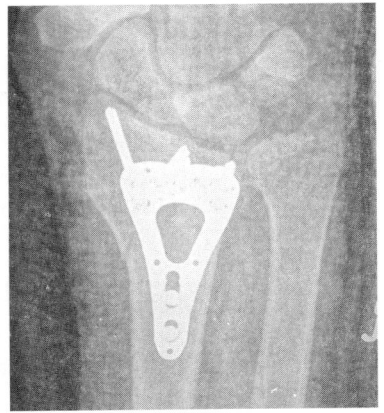

Figure 7.5 Volar open reduction with plate for unstable, higher-energy wrist fracture

- open injuries
- intra-articular displacement
- lots of fragments (comminution)
- poor bone quality (reduction will collapse)
- palmarly displaced/angulated fractures (slip more frequently; malunions poorly tolerated by patients)

Fractures with any, or a combination, of these characteristics need to be treated more aggressively from the outset with more robust reduction/fixation techniques.

Classification System

These basic principles should guide us to a useful classification system for wrist fractures. There is no perfect system, and there are many eponyms in common usage regarding wrist injuries, which can be confusing.

COMMON EPONYMS OF WRIST INJURIES

Colles' fracture
- extra-articular; dorsally angulated/displaced metaphyseal fracture in adults (actually described before the advent of X-rays)

Smith's fracture
- extra-articular; volarly angulated/displaced metaphyseal fracture

Volar Barton's fracture
- intra-articular fracture where the volar lip of the distal radius is displaced volarly

Chauffeur's fracture
- intra-articular fracture of the radial styloid

Galeazzi fracture/dislocation
- high-energy injury; volarly angulated distal radius fracture with dorsal dislocation of distal ulna; DRUJ disrupted

Die punch fracture
- intra-articular impaction fracture of lunate bone into distal radius

---

To avoid confusion, it is probably best just to **describe the fracture in terms of the following**:

- displaced or nondisplaced
- extra-articular or intra-articular (very important)
- dorsal or volar angulation/displacement
- number of major fragments
  - 2 = extra-articular
  - 3 = intra-articular (lunate area)
  - 4 = coronal split; 4 +

- any dislocations
  - between distal radius and ulna (DRUJ)?
  - within the carpal bones? (Look for the lunate; the space between all carpal bones should be equal.)

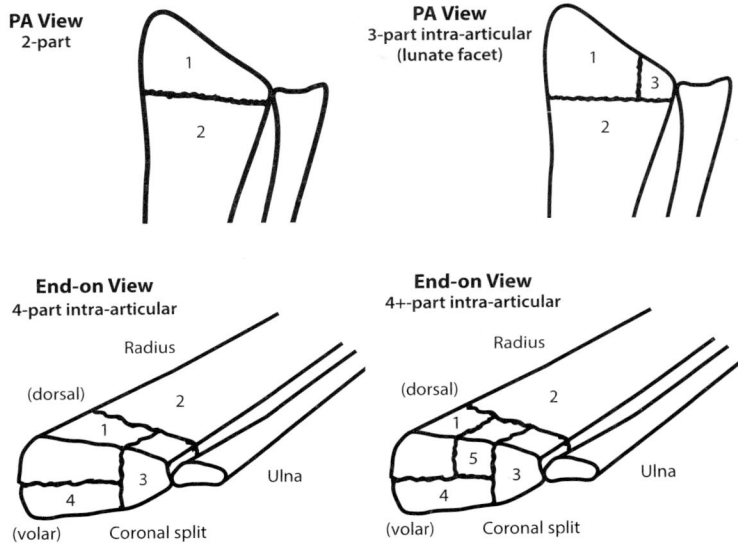

Figure 7.6 Diagram demonstrating increasing number of carpal fragments as energy increases

Emergency Room Treatment

First, ensure there are no small, open wounds. These are typically puncture wounds at the apex of the angulatory deformity (volar wrist in a Colles' type fracture). These are seen if the skin is very thin in elderly women or in horrendously crooked deformities. Often, the wound is from the distal ulna, not the radius! Note the wound location, cover with a sterile gauze, and then splint the extremity.

Since there is often a great deal of swelling, temporary below-elbow splints are the preferred way to immobilize the wrist rather than a cast. Even if you do a closed reduction before the patient leaves the E.R., either use a custom-moulded dorsal splint or a cast that is univalved to allow for swelling.

If the injury cannot be dealt with by closed reduction in the emergency department, it still needs to be splinted before transfer. As in ankle fractures, the wrist should be realigned before splinting if there is pressure on the soft tissues or circulation compromise to the fingers. Any return to a more normal alignment will help — the X-ray does not have to be perfect!

TIMING FOR FOLLOW-UP

For a stable, low-energy fracture pattern reduced in the E.R.:

- see in clinic within 7–10 days
- re-X-ray
- replace splint or univalved cast with full below-elbow cast
- if reduction slips → refer

TIMING FOR SURGERY

For an unstable fracture pattern:

- well-aligned; soft tissues okay = < 10 days
- not fully reduced; soft tissues at risk = < 24 hours
- open wound = < 6 hours

Operative Treatment

The principles of wrist fracture operative treatment include the following:

- radius out to length (styloid tip 1 cm distal to ulna)
- distal radius joint space perfect
- neutral sagittal alignment or better (N = 12 degrees volar tilt)
- no volar translation of carpus (very unstable situation)
- DRUJ reduced and stable
- avoid above-elbow immobilization (very bad in adults for stiffness)
- cast no longer than 6 weeks
- allow early finger and elbow motion

We try to achieve these goals in a *graduated manner of complexity* depending on the previously mentioned risk factors for instability of the fracture regarding the energy level involved in producing it.

Treatment for Specific Fractures

LOW-ENERGY FRACTURES

SIMPLE DORSALLY ANGULATED FRACTURES

- closed reduction/below-elbow cast (can be done in E.R.)
- add percutaneous pins (if done in the O.R.)

MEDIUM-ENERGY FRACTURES

EXTRA-ARTICULAR, MORE DISPLACED FRACTURES

- closed reduction/percutaneous pins

Fortunately, the previous two groups probably make up 80% of wrist fractures.

SCAPHOID FRACTURES

This is a common injury in the 18- to 25-year-old male population. Diagnosis can be tricky early on. Splint and re-X-ray in 2 weeks if in doubt.

- fracture can be in waist, proximal pole, or distal pole
- below-elbow thumb spica cast for 8–12 weeks = 90% heal
- early ORIF better if
  - greater than 2 mm displaced or flexed (DISI) high-demand occupation (decrease casting)

- increased nonunion if[1]
  - more than 1 month delay in onset of treatment
  - proximal pole fractures
  - greater than 2 mm displacement or scaphoid flexed
  - noncompliant patients and smokers

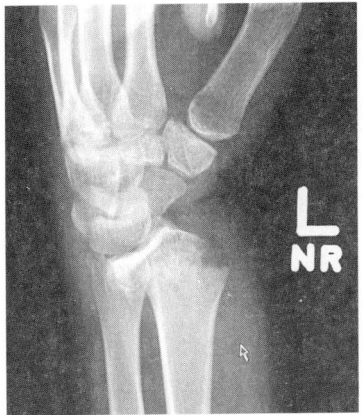

Figure 7.7 Medium-energy extra-articular wrist fracture

HIGHER-ENERGY FRACTURES

INTRA-ARTICULAR, LARGE FRAGMENTS

- ORIF with plates (usually volar)
- about 10–15% of fractures

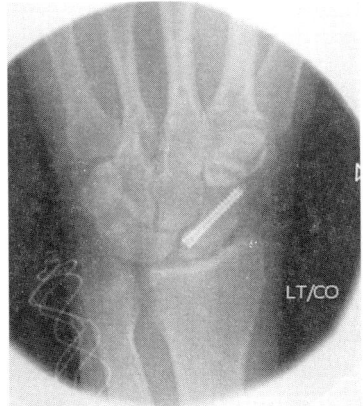

Figure 7.8 Scaphoid fracture fixation screw

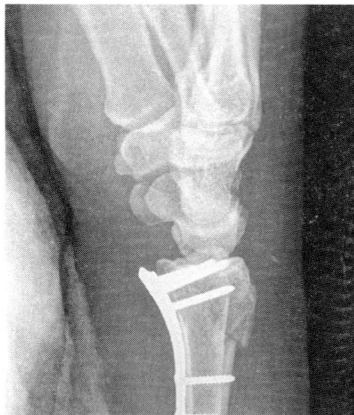

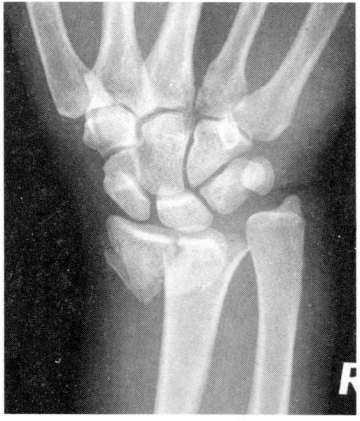

Figure 7.9 Higher-energy distal radius fracture treated with locking plates

Figure 7.10 Highest-energy fracture (Note the large amount of fracture displacement and intra-articular extension.)

HIGHEST-ENERGY FRACTURES

COMMINUTED/INTRA-ARTICULAR

- locked plates?
- add external fixation devices?
- add pins?
- delayed bone grafting?

CARPAL FRACTURE/DISLOCATIONS

- ORIF with pins/ligament repairs; or plates
- rare, but always difficult to treat

Outcomes

The outcome will depend on both fracture-specific parameters and patient-specific characteristics.

Fracture-Specific Parameters

The biggest factor will be whether this was a low- or high-energy injury (just as in every other region of the MSK). More displacement, comminution, and soft tissue damage means more swelling of the fingers and hand and more stiffness later on.

- intra-articular involvement → predicts more joint stiffness/possible osteoarthritis

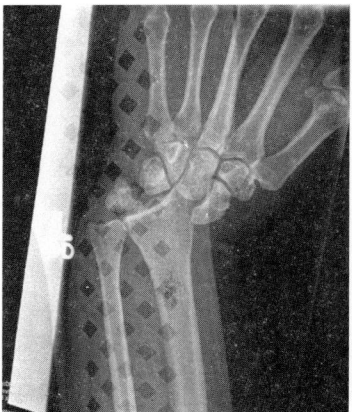

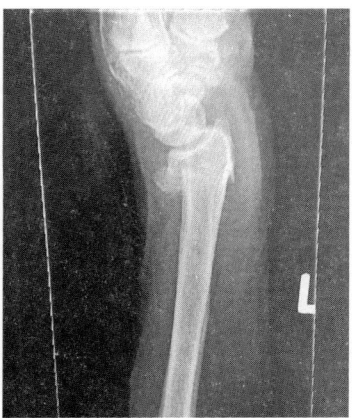

Figure 7.11 Carpal fracture/dislocation: Look for the lunate. (It is still in its usual location while remainder of the carpal bones have been dislocated!)

Figure 7.12 Common loss of reduction seen in poor bone: functional result can still be good.

- poor bone quality/osteoporosis → predicts loss of reduction/ shortening

However, there is one exception: just because an extra-articular distal radius fracture has collapsed and shortened, it will not necessarily mean a bad result, particularly in an older patient with a dorsally angulated malunion.

Patient-Specific Characteristics

Certain factors predict a good outcome and others predict problems.

GOOD PREDICTORS:

- older, more sedentary patients (do not mind the cosmetic bump on their wrists)
- good-quality bone (will help any fracture hold together while healing)
- happy people who get on with their busy lives (and move their fingers while in their casts)

POTENTIAL PROBLEMS:

- WCB injuries (take much longer to heal and return to work than noncompensation cases)
- anxious/injury-focused patients
  - These patients (statistically likely to be women) are at risk for developing RSDS (reflex sympathetic dystrophy syndrome).

- This can be a very disabling complication involving the whole upper limb (swelling, stiffness, pain).
- Treatment is early recognition, physician encouragement, and LOTS of physiotherapy.

REFERENCE

1. Ring D, Jupiter JB, Herndon JH. Acute fractures of the scaphoid. *J Am Acad Orthop Surg.* 2000;8(4):225–31. Medline:10951111

8

Knee

Knee injuries round off the top four common MSK injuries that present to the emergency department/orthopaedic surgeon.

Soft Tissue Injuries

Soft tissue injuries of the knee are probably more common than bony injuries, particularly in adults younger than 60 years of age. The weak links around the skeletally mature knee are the ligaments, joint capsule, and menisci. The bone is strong and does not generally fracture until osteoporosis becomes prevalent in the more elderly age group. These are generally low- to medium-energy injuries. In high-energy injuries, just as in any area of the MSK, the weak link principle may not apply, and any fracture combination can occur (even through strong bone).

Locked Knee

This is a very common presentation to the emergency department. Typically, the patient has had a several-month history of intermittent catching or partial locking of the affected knee, which suddenly will not unlock. Usually, the patient has been squatting or kneeling and is unable to extend the knee fully in attempting to get up.

The physical exam shows an inability to fully weight bear, medial joint-line tenderness, and active ROM decrease. (There is always a block to full extension, but flexion may be > 90 degrees.)

There are two subgroups:

- *young adults* = bucket handle tear medial meniscus; normal knee X-ray
- *middle-aged* = degenerative meniscal debris; look for early O/A X-ray changes

TREATMENT

Most of these locked knees will unlock on their own, particularly in the degenerative knee age group, over a few days. Use crutches, NSAID, and gentle ROM in warm bath water.

Ultimately, an arthroscopy will solve the problem — the timing depends on the response to conservative measures and the likely diagnosis. Bucket-handle meniscal tears in young people should be done within 2 weeks; degenerative debris tears can be done in weeks or even months.

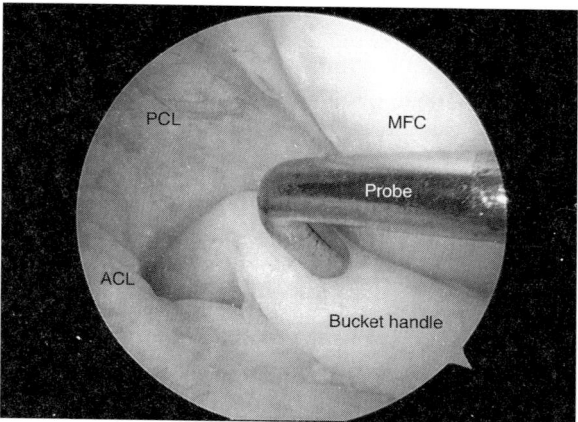

Figure 8.1 Bucket-handle tear of meniscus

Arthroscopic treatment consists of excision of the meniscal tear. Ninety percent of these are medial meniscal, except in the ACL-deficient knee where the lateral meniscus can tear. Occasionally, the tear is amenable to repair in the younger patient. The status of the ACL is important in this decision.

Knee Strain

A knee strain can be described clinically as a medial collateral ligament (MCL) injury, or less commonly, a lateral collateral ligament (LCL)/posterior capsular strain situation. These are very common low- or medium-energy soft tissue injuries. Typically, the knee is twisted, often into valgus, and the patient falls down. Generally, the patient limps but can still walk, as the knee is not grossly unstable. There is a slow onset of swelling over a few hours.

The physical exam shows localized tenderness and swelling over the medial (or lateral) joint line/insertion of the collateral ligaments. Gentle valgus or varus testing (with the knee flexed about 10 degrees) will show increased opening of the joint, compared to the contralateral, normal knee.

Injuries are generally graded as follows:

I = tenderness, no joint opening

II = abnormal opening with end point

III = joint opens; no end point

Plain X-rays should be normal; look for avulsion fractures from the fibular head in lateral collateral ligament/posterior capsule injuries.

TREATMENT

- Grade I = symptomatic; no bracing necessary
- Grades II and III = crutches; partial weight bearing; extension knee brace for 2–3 weeks; then physiotherapy and hinged knee brace for 6–8 weeks

Surgical repair is generally not indicated for an isolated MCL or LCL tear unless the patient is noncompliant with bracing, the knee is more unstable than expected (posterior capsular tear + MCL or LCL), or a repairable bony avulsion fracture is present.

Knee Blowout

A knee blowout can be described clinically as an injury of the ACL, ACL/MCL, or ACL/MCL/medial meniscus. These are higher-energy and more dramatic injuries than the knee sprains. They are seen in running, skiing, and many other aggressive sports where the planted knee is twisted and extended at the same time. Patients often feel a "pop" in their knee and experience immediate severe pain. Generally, the knee *swells within minutes*, and because the knee feels so unstable, they cannot walk. These patients usually present to the emergency department earlier than the knee strain group.

The physical exam shows impressive knee swelling, limited active knee motion, but an intact straight leg lift (extensor mechanism is intact). Ligament integrity should be compared to the contralateral knee, which is examined first, partially to gain the patient's confidence. Look for the following:

- collateral ligaments: gently check for abnormal opening and end points

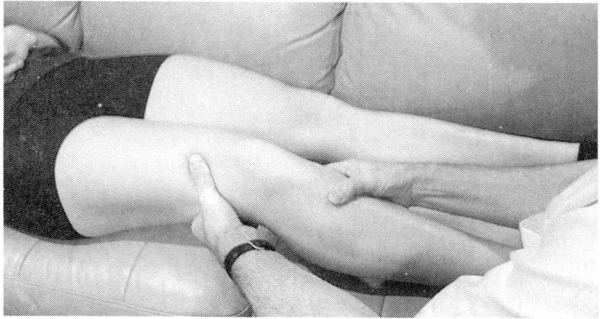

Figure 8.2 Lachman test

- anterior cruciate ligament:
  - Lachman test can be done gently, even on a swollen knee; look for increased translation and lack of an end point
  - anterior drawer test: more difficult to do in acute trauma situation

Plain X-rays should be ordered to rule out fractures or bony avulsions. Look particularly at the tibial spine area.

> Ligament integrity should be compared to the contralateral knee, examined first to gain the patient's confidence.

TREATMENT

GENERAL

- Do not aspirate the knee (unless it is agonizingly tense, which is rare).
- Splint the knee in an extension brace; crutches; partial weight bearing.
- Early ROM at home is allowed.
- Review in 1–2 weeks.
- Re-examine when the knee is less swollen and painful.

SPECIFIC TREATMENT

This is where the controversy exists in the literature: who needs an urgent MRI, who should have early surgery, and if so, what kind?[1]

Important factors to consider include the following:

- age and activity level of the patient (younger; more active)
- isolated ACL or a combined injury (Is the knee so grossly unstable that early ROM is impossible?)

- block to knee extension at 2 weeks (torn meniscus?)
- bony avulsion fracture: should be fixed if large enough
- high-performance athlete?

If any of these factors are present, an MRI should be done early. If gross instability or ROM blockage is the problem, consideration for an early EUA in the O.R. for MCL repair, with or without arthroscopy, is an option for any community-based orthopaedic surgeon.

These days, most large hospitals have a sports medicine orthopaedic surgeon who specializes in ACL repair. Certainly, the high-performance athletes and patients with more complicated combined knee injuries should be referred to these surgeons as soon as a firm diagnosis can be made.

In the lower-demand patient, and the patients who are improving at 1 to 2 weeks, start physiotherapy with increasing weight bearing in a hinged brace. An elective MRI and possible referral for ACL reconstruction can be made weeks or months later.

MCL tears heal without surgery in a brace, but complete ACL tears do not. Even if the ACL is repaired end-to-end primarily, it will fail. ACL surgery is, therefore, of the reconstruction type, where a donor tendon is tunneled into the ACL site. Most surgery of this type is done many months, or even years, after the original injury. Exceptions to this are usually in the higher-demand, combined ligament/meniscal patient group. However, many lower-demand patients will function quite nicely with an ACL-deficient knee and never need referral for reconstruction. Many of these injuries turn out to be partial tears of the ACL, which also do not need to be reconstructed.

In summary, for knee blowout, the following are goals of treatment:

- early diagnosis
- splint until stable
- early protected ROM

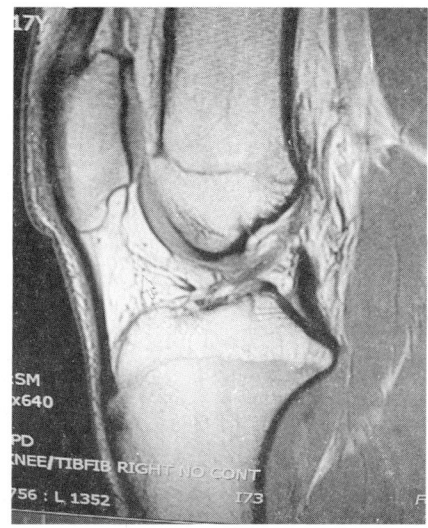

Figure 8.3 ACL tear on MRI

Perform surgery if the following:

- grossly unstable knee
- block to motion
- bony avulsion fracture
- high-performance athlete

Locked knee, knee strain, and knee blowout are the most commonly seen soft tissue injuries around the knee and should be familiar to all primary-care doctors.

For completeness, there are two less common, but still important, soft tissue injuries around the knee: (a) extensor mechanism failures and (b) frank knee dislocations.

Extensor Mechanism Failures

Extensor mechanism failures include both quadriceps and patellar tendon tears. The extensor mechanism can fail with a displaced patellar fracture, which is easy to diagnose, but it can also fail through the soft tissues. The knee is diffusely swollen and tender, usually after a fall on the flexed knee, or knee that is actively extending while falling.

The **hallmark for diagnosis** is an **inability to extend the knee actively against gravity**. X-rays show no fractures but may show either a high riding or low patella.

Try to palpate a soft tissue defect either above (quadriceps tear) or below (patellar tendon tear) the patellar. Quadriceps ruptures are more common in older men and in heavily muscled body builders. Patellar tendon injuries are more common in younger patients.

If the patient cannot actively raise the leg into a straight position, treatment is surgical. Try to repair these within 2 weeks of the injury. The defect is repaired with sutures; sometimes the tendon needs to be reanchored to the avulsion site with wires or screws.

These are serious injuries and rehabilita-

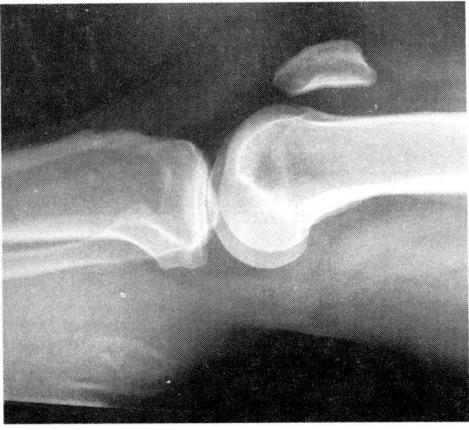

Figure 8.4 Patellar tendon rupture with patellar alta

tion is significant: 3 months on average. Knee stiffness, extensor lag, and DVT are common complications. It is better to heal a fractured patella than to heal an extensor soft tissue tear!

Knee Dislocation

True knee dislocations occur at the femoral–tibial articulation and do not include isolated patellar dislocations. These are rare injuries, fortunately, since they are always hard to treat and are fraught with complications. For the tibia to dislocate on the femur, by definition, most of the soft tissue constraints around the knee must be torn (ACL, PCL, MCL, menisci, post/lateral corner).

Two presentations are seen: (a) in the context of a high-energy, multiple injury (motor vehicle accident [MVA], etc.) and (b) as a lower-energy iso-

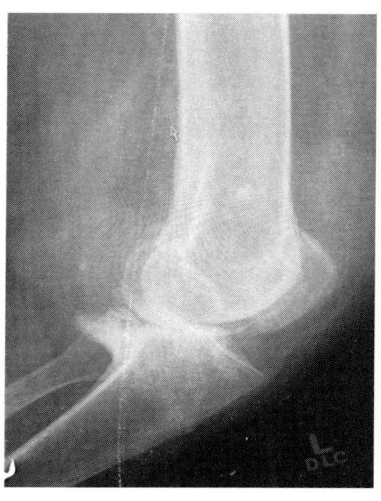

Figure 8.5 Anterior near dislocation of tibia on femur (lower-energy subtype)

lated knee injury in a morbidly obese patient, usually with lax ligaments. Close follow-up by an orthopaedic surgeon is essential in both groups.

The dislocation needs to be reduced, and kept reduced, within 6 hours. This should be done in the O.R., ideally under general anaesthetic. The knee will be grossly unstable postreduction, so splinting, external fixation, or partial early ligament repair will

> Watch out for associated injuries to the common peroneal nerve and/or the popliteal vessels — especially in high-energy injuries.

be required after reduction. Basically, enough of the ligaments and soft tissues are repaired early, to get the knee moving, and reconstructions are done later.

In the high-energy group, imaging to look for partial tears of the popliteal vessels (digital angiography, Doppler studies, etc.) should be ordered after the knee joint is reduced and stabilized, as late aneurysms can develop and can be missed early on.[2]

These are bad injuries, even without the neurovascular complications. With this amount of soft tissue injury, the knee can become either chronically stiff (higher-energy group) or weak and unstable (obese lower-energy group). Vascular injuries can be repaired early with good results. Peroneal nerve injuries have an unpredictable prognosis, and treatment varies on the nature of the actual injury to the nerve itself.

Bony Injuries

Bony knee injuries are quite common and can be broadly classified as (a) those that occur in healthy people with good bone and (b) those that occur in the elderly (or in osteoporotic bone).

KNEE FRACTURES IN GOOD BONE	KNEE FRACTURES IN OSTEOPOROTIC BONE
• patellar fractures	• low-energy tibial plateau fractures
• medium- to high-energy tibial plateau fractures	• low-energy distal femur fractures; often around TKR implant
• high-energy distal femur fractures	

Fractures in Good Bone

Fractures in healthy bone consist of (a) patellar fractures, (b) medium- to high-energy tibial plateau fractures, and (c) high-energy distal femur fractures.

PATELLAR FRACTURES

These occur, in all ages, with a fall or contusion directly onto the flexed knee/patella. Diagnosis is easy on X-ray. The degree of comminution varies with the energy level of the injury.

Minimally displaced fractures (< 2 mm distraction), with intact active knee extension against gravity, can be treated conservatively in a splint and then physiotherapy. Displaced fractures should be surgically repaired. Patellectomy is rarely indicated.

Postoperative problems include knee stiffness, extensor lag, O/A of the patellofemoral joint, and metal fixation prominence around the subcutaneous patella (elective wire removal commonly needed).

MEDIUM- TO HIGH-ENERGY TIBIAL PLATEAU FRACTURES

The tibial plateau is strong in healthy adults, so fractures are usually not low-energy injuries (in contrast to plateau fractures in the elderly). They are seen in skiing and sports injuries and in MVAs.

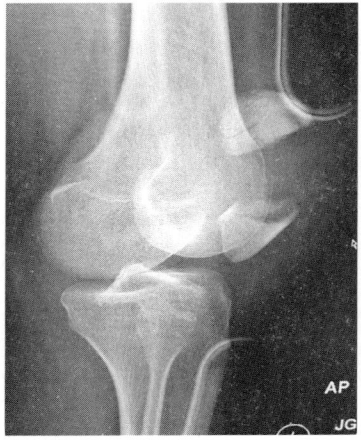

Figure 8.6 Displaced patellar fracture

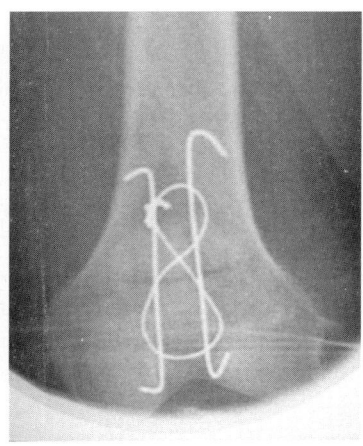

Figure 8.7 ORIF of patellar fracture

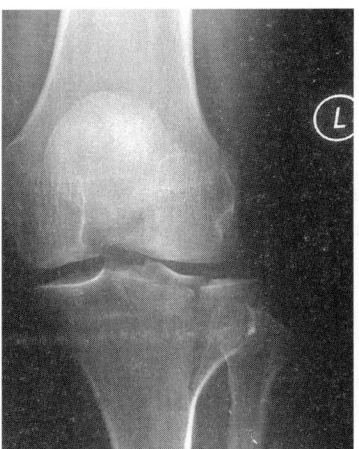

Figure 8.8 Schatzker Type I tibial plateau fracture

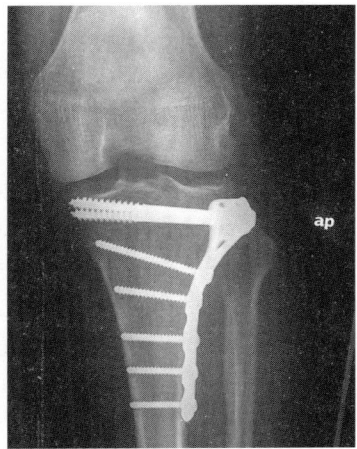

Figure 8.9 ORIF tibial plateau fracture

The Schatzker ASIF classification is widely used.[3] Lateral plateau fractures (I–III) are the most common and are generally straightforward to fix; medial plateau fractures (IV) are higher energy, tip into varus, and are very hard to fix. Bicondylar (V) and more complex patterns (VI) are high-energy injuries with high complication rates.

These fractures do quite well if they are in the lateral plateau and a good ORIF is achieved. The IV to VI group can be very challenging to fix because of problems of residual varus, joint stiffness, neurovascular issues, and premature osteoarthritis. Primary-care doctors must be on the lookout for neurovascular injuries and compartment syndromes — particularly in the higher-energy injuries.

HIGH-ENERGY DISTAL FEMUR FRACTURES

Distal femur fractures are very serious and, fortunately, not that common. They require very high energy to break healthy, strong bone around the knee. They are seen in motorcycle, car, and industrial accidents. Look for associated injuries around the knee and elsewhere.

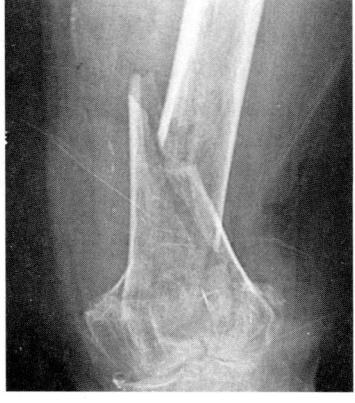

Fractures are often intra-articular and plating or retrograde nailing is required. Knee motion is usually never the same and osteoarthritis is a complication.

Figure 8.10 Comminuted distal femur fracture

Fractures in Osteoporotic Bone

Osteoporotic bone fractures come in two varieties: (a) low-energy tibial plateau fractures and (b) low-energy distal femur fractures, often around TKR implant.

LOW-ENERGY TIBIAL PLATEAU FRACTURES

Tibial plateau fractures are common injuries in the elderly. The metaphyseal area of the proximal tibia becomes the weak link around the knee, and the plateau fractures easily with any angulatory (usually valgus) stress on the knee. The result is a lateral tibial plateau fracture, usually minimally displaced (Schatzker Type II or III) due to bone compaction.

Many of these fractures can be treated conservatively unless a significant step (> 5 mm) is present in the joint on a plain X-ray or CT scan, or unless the valgus exceeds 5 degrees.

Conservative treatment includes non- or feather-weight bearing in a splint or brace for 4 weeks and then gradual increased weight bearing and physiotherapy for 4–8 weeks. In this age group, slight joint irregularity or mild valgus can be treated once the fracture has healed with a primary total knee replacement semi-electively.

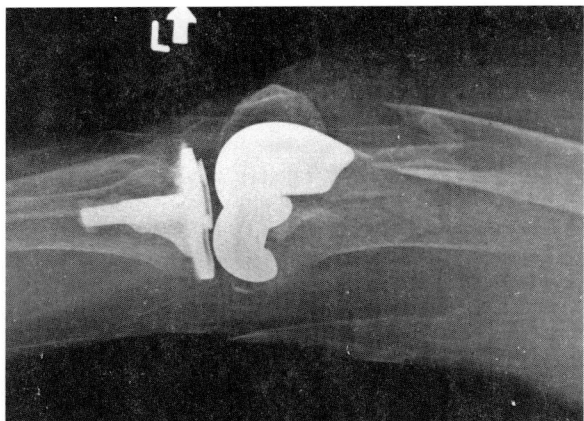

Figure 8.11 Fractured femur above TKR implant

LOW-ENERGY DISTAL FEMUR FRACTURES

Distal femur fractures are common low-energy injuries seen in older patients with osteoporotic bone and knee replacements. They are becoming more common because so many more people are walking around with hip and knee replacements. They are particularly common in rheumatoid arthritis patients.

Typically, patients experience a slow, twisting fall. The joint implant acts as a stress riser, and a peri-prosthetic fracture results in the weak bone around the implant. Alternately, a patient with a stiff, nonreplaced arthritic knee can sustain a supracondylar fracture of the femur.

Treatment is usually surgical and can be quite challenging since there is not a lot of bone to work with. Various forms of locking plates are usually used. The implant is only revised if it has been chronically loose.

PERI-PROSTHETIC HIP FRACTURES

Although not located around the knee, these fractures are very similar to peri-prosthetic knee fractures in origin and treatment. A pure dislocation of the THR is much more common after a fall than a peri-prosthetic fracture overall. However, they do occur, particularly if the patient lands on the lateral side of the hip.

Again, the hip implant stem acts as a stress riser, and the femur breaks at the distal tip of the implant and then spirals proximally

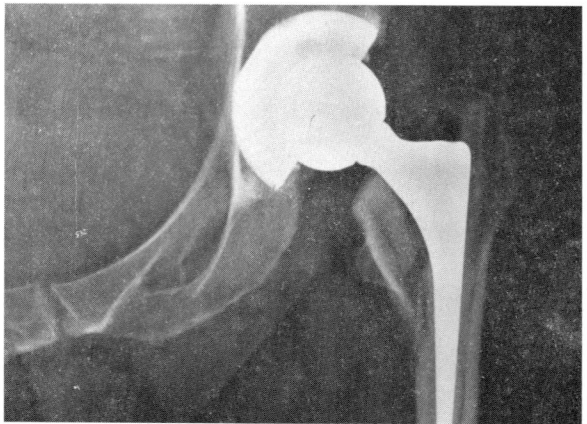

Figure 8.12 X-ray of peri-prosthetic THR fracture (Note fracture around femoral stem.)

(usually). It is very important to determine if the hip replacement was chronically painful with loosening before the injury. If obviously loose, then the stem should be revised; if not loose, then the fracture is usually wired/plated.

Isolated fractures of the greater or lesser trochanter, in a patient with a THR, can usually be treated conservatively if the femoral stem is not loose.

REFERENCES

1. Hantes ME, Tsarouhas A. Timing of ACL surgery: Any evidence? In: Siebold R, Dejour D, Zaffagnini S, editors. Anterior cruciate ligament reconstruction: A practical surgical guide. Springer; 2014. p. 123–7.

2. Stannard JP, Sheils TM, Lopez-Ben RR, McGwin Jr G, Robinson JT, Volgas DA. Vascular injuries in knee dislocations: the role of physical examination in determining the need for arteriography. *J. Bone Joint Am.* 2004;86(5):910–5.

3. Walton NP, Harish S, Roberts C, Blundell C. AO or Schatzker? How reliable is classification of tibial plateau fractures? *Arch Orthop Trauma Surg.* 2003;123(8):396–8. http://dx.doi.org/10.1007/s00402-003-0573-1. Medline:14574596

9

Shoulder

The shoulder is commonly injured in falls and in numerous sporting activities. The type of injury, or the weak link, can be predicted by the age of the patient and the amount of energy involved in the injury. There are two main age groups where these injuries are common: older teenagers/young adults and the elderly.

CHECKLIST OF COMMON SHOULDER INJURIES
AFTER A FALL, RELATED TO AGE

Young children
• mid-shaft clavicle fractures

Older children
• Salter II proximal humerus fractures

Young adults/older teenagers
• shoulder dislocations
• AC joint separations
• clavicle fractures

Middle-aged adults
• proximal humerus fractures (Many are unstable patterns.)

Elderly adults
• impacted, stable proximal humerus fractures

Children's shoulder injuries are described in detail in Chapter 19. Although common, these injuries do very well, and remodelling around the shoulder is significant.

Young Adults/Older Teenagers with Closed Growth Plates

This age group is commonly seen in the emergency department because they are so active in sports (and are often high-risk takers).

Although their bones are strong, the forces involved are usually high, so the fractures and deformities can be quite impressive. The problem with this group of patients is compliance; the injury is often not allowed sufficient time to heal and the return to sports is premature. This often leads to problems with recurrent instability or nonunions.

In contrast, in older adults/the elderly, the major problem after shoulder injuries is stiffness. This should be kept in mind when treating shoulder injuries in the different age groups.

Shoulder Dislocations

Shoulder dislocations are discussed, in general terms, in Chapter 3 and Chapter 28, under urgent orthopaedic conditions, regarding principles of reduction.

Dislocation is a common sports injury and found mostly in young people. These young people have strong bones and fused growth plates, so the weak link is often the joint capsule.

Classification is useful and important:

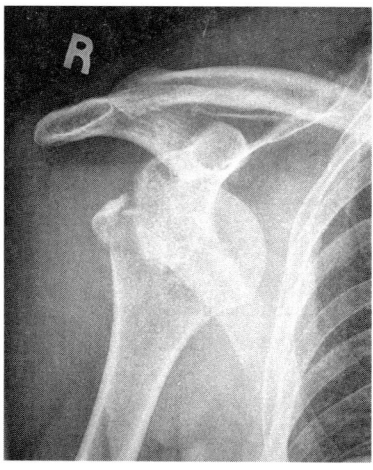

Figure 9.1 Anterior shoulder dislocation (with small greater tuberosity fragment)

- acute/traumatic versus atraumatic/habitual
- direction: anterior (90%) > posterior > inferior – multidirectional

ACUTE UNIDIRECTIONAL DISLOCATIONS

Most cases that present to the emergency department are young males with an acute, unidirectional shoulder dislocation (90% are anterior dislocations). They have a history of a fall or a blow to the shoulder with the shoulder abducted and externally rotated. Generally, they are unable to reduce the dislocation at the scene and are brought to the E.R. with their arm adducted across their chest. The axillary nerve can be stretched, so check for numbness in the lateral deltoid area, pre-reduction. Good X-rays in two planes confirm the diagnosis. (AP and trans-scapular lateral X-ray can be done without moving the painful shoulder.)

Posterior and inferior dislocations are much less common than anterior, subcoracoid dislocations. Posterior dislocations classically present late (days or weeks) after a grand-mal seizure (where the shoulder has been violently internally rotated and pops out the back of the capsule). They can also occur after a direct blow to the front of the shoulder with the arm abducted. Inferior dislocations are rare and occur only if the arm is injured in full elevation over the patient's head.

Treatment is gentle closed reduction in the emergency department. The key to reduction, regardless of specific technique, is adequate muscle relaxation. This often involves enough sedation to limit adequate ventilation post-reduction, so plan ahead and have a second person to monitor breathing.

Once reduced, these patients need to be placed in a shoulder immobilizer and followed closely for the first 6 weeks. The shoulder immobilizer is worn 23 hours per day for the first 2 weeks and then physiotherapy is started. Sports and activities are gradually reintroduced over 3 months. The capsule will heal provided there is no repeat injury in the first 3 months. Recurrent dislocation problems are directly related to compliance during this period.

Historically, surgery is only indicated for recurrent traumatic dislocations, often "three strikes and you're out." Various operations exist to reconstruct the shoulder capsule and its restraining structures. Many of these procedures can now be performed arthroscopically.

There is a trend among sports medicine specialists to be more aggressive in first-time dislocators and proceed straight to MRI and surgery, especially in high-performance athletes.[1] In this patient subpopulation, a telephone call for early orthopaedic advice may be prudent.

MULTIDIRECTIONAL/HABITUAL DISLOCATIONS

Multidirectional/Habitual dislocations are more commonly seen in the office setting and in young women. A good history for an initial injury is usually absent, and the shoulder pops and clicks (and partially subluxes in various positions). These patients have ligamentous laxity in all their joints (check their fingers).

Treatment is nonsurgical: physiotherapy and chronic exercises to strengthen the shoulder girdle. Surgery has a high recurrence rate.

Acromio-Clavicular (AC) Joint Injuries

These are common injuries in young adults after a fall on the point of the shoulder. They are common cycling, rugby, and hockey injuries. Presentation is classic, with an obvious painful step at the AC joint area.

Classification is useful: only the Grade III or higher injuries ever require surgery (clavicle > 100% displaced on acromion).

Most of these injuries can be treated conservatively, with a shoulder immobilizer for 1–2 weeks, and then physiotherapy, with a slow return to sports over weeks/months.

Surgery is generally reserved for high-grade injuries with marked displacement, or cosmetically ugly deformities in thin patients, and is done more frequently in the dominant arm of men who perform heavy labour. Consultation with an orthopaedic surgeon is often wise in borderline cases.

Fortunately, most AC injuries are Type II or Type III with only mild deformities.

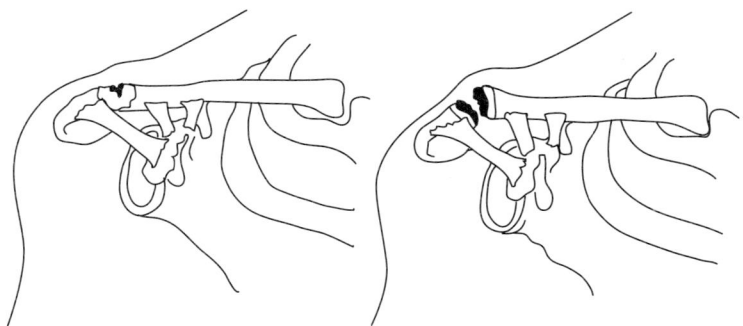

Type I = AC ligament strain   Type II = AC ligament torn

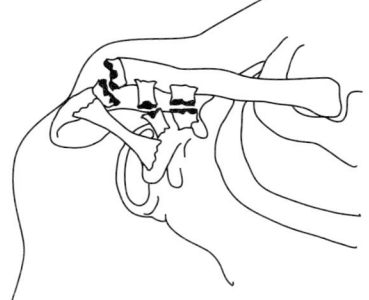

Type III = AC and CC ligaments torn

Figure 9.2 Simplified AC joint injury classification

Clavicle Fractures

Clavicle fractures are seen in young males typically after a high-energy blow to the shoulder area (falls off motorcycles, all-terrain vehicles, etc.). Generally, the clavicle fractures in the middle third. Historically, these have been treated conservatively, in the same manner as AC joint injuries.

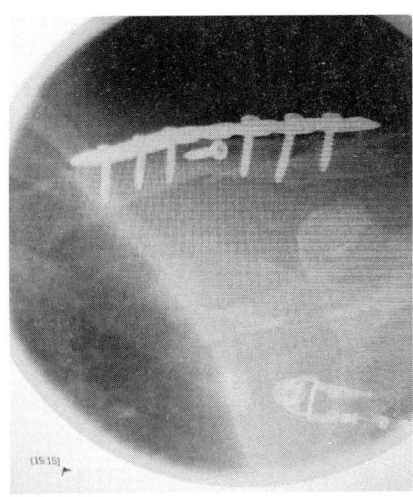

Figure 9.3 ORIF of left clavicle for unstable fracture pattern

There is a trend, particularly among recently trained orthopaedic surgeons, to treat more of these surgically, with plating. This is particularly true in fractures associated with a higher nonunion rate initially.[2] Risk factors for potential nonunion include the following:

- displacement > 150% shaft width of clavicle
- comminuted shaft fracture
- subcutaneous bone fragments
- dominant arm in labourers

Proximal Humerus Fractures

Middle-Aged Patients

Shoulder fractures are not particularly common in middle-aged people. Unfortunately, because their bone is reasonably good, higher energy is required to break the bone and unstable fracture patterns often occur. Contrarily, in elderly patients, most of these fractures are low energy through poor bone and fracture patterns are stable.

Classification of proximal humerus fractures is very predictive of treatment. Dr. Neer's system — based on four fragments around the shoulder — is widely used and should be learned:

- a fragment is only "counted"
  - if it is angulated > 45 degrees
  - if it is displaced > 1 cm

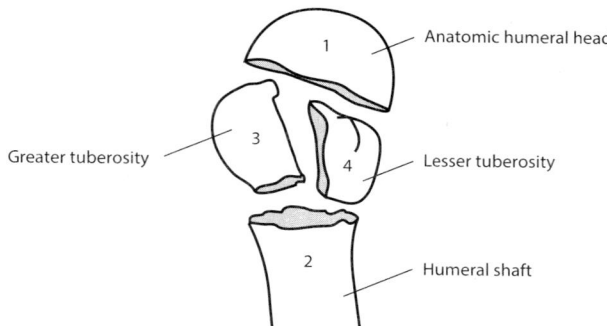

Figure 9.4 Four-part humerus fracture

Proximal humerus fractures follow a predictable continuum from stable/low energy/impacted to more unstable patterns with two or more fragments. The most unstable fractures are associated with a dislocation as well. The risk of AVN and nonunion increases with the number of fragments. Treatment is ultimately determined by the age of the patient, quality of the bone, and the Neer classification.

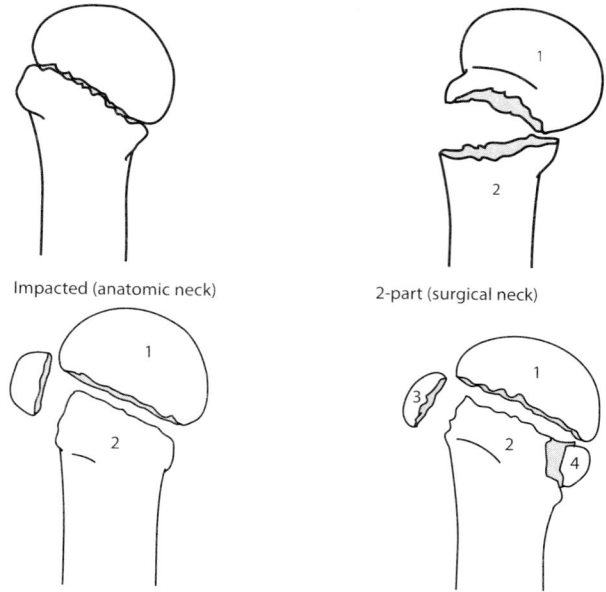

Figure 9.5 Neer classification of proximal humerus fractures (modified). All fractures + or - a dislocation.

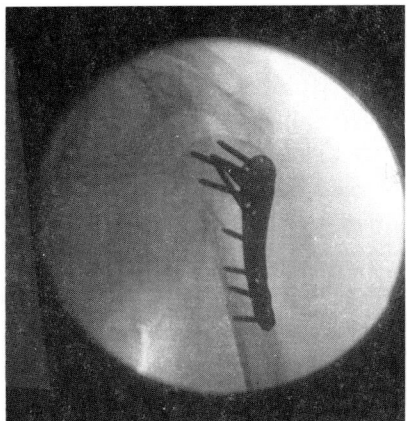 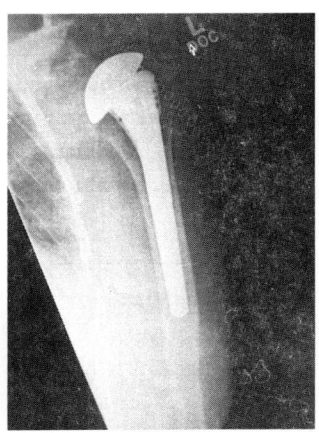

Figure 9.6 ORIF of unstable 2-part unstable proximal humerus fracture

Figure 9.7 Hemi-arthroplasty for 4+ fragment proximal humerus fracture

Good-quality AP and trans-scapular lateral X-rays will usually show an unstable two or more fragment fracture pattern immediately. A CT scan of the shoulder can be helpful if the joint is involved.

Surgical treatment should be done early if an unstable pattern is present. Options for surgery include the following:

- closed reduction/pinning (some 2-part fractures)
- formal ORIF with screws/plates (if bone is good)
  - most unstable fractures treated this way

- hemi-arthroplasty of head
  - in 4+ fragments with poor bone; AVN

Postoperative physiotherapy is very important in these patients, as stiffness is an immense problem in any older patient with a shoulder fracture (with or without surgery).

Elderly Patients

Elderly patients make up one of the largest groups seen with shoulder fractures. These are low-energy injuries in poor osteoporotic bone; fortunately, most of these fractures are impacted or stable. More than 90% can be treated conservatively.

Typically, the fracture occurs at the anatomic neck/metaphyseal junction and, according to the Neer classification, is rarely displaced more than 1 cm, so functionally, these are one-part/impacted fractures. Rarely (< 10%), there are three or more fragments that are functionally displaced and, because of poor bone, these may be candidates for early hemi-arthroplasty. Even then, many low-demand and elderly patients will do well with conservative treatment.

A few points about **conservative treatment of proximal humerus fractures** are warranted because the details are important.

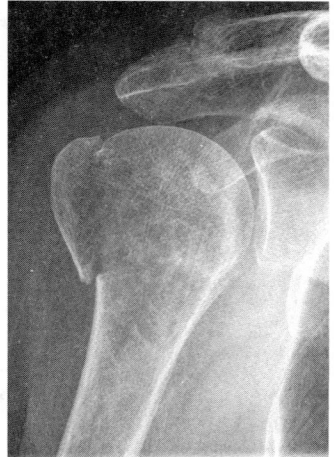

Figure 9.8 Three-fragment proximal humerus fracture in poor bone

- Place the arm in a high-quality shoulder immobilizer before discharge (not just a simple sling; good arm support is essential for good pain relief).
- Instruct the patient to sleep propped up on pillows or in a reclining chair for the first 2 weeks.
- Instruct the patient to remove the immobilizer 2–3 times per day for gentle elbow motion exercises, armpit care, and bathing; gentle pendulum exercises of the shoulder while standing are helpful. Elderly patients will leave the immobilizer untouched for 2 weeks unless you instruct them otherwise!
- Tell the patient to expect elbow/hand swelling and bruising.
- See the patient again in 10–14 days for re-X-ray and referral to physiotherapy.
- Wean the shoulder immobilizer over 3–4 weeks; gentle ROM only; no weights allowed; physiotherapy for 3 months.
- Three months for fracture healing.
- Expect some shoulder stiffness. (Few return to normal overhead motion.)

REFERENCES

1. Jakobsen BW, Johannsen HV, Suder P, et al. Primary repair versus conservative treatment of first-time traumatic anterior dislocation of the shoulder: a randomized study with 10-year follow-up. *Arthroscopy: The Journal of Arthroscopic and Related Surgery.* 2007;23(2):118–23. http://dx.doi.org/10.1016/j.arthro.2006.11.004.

2. Kim W, McKee M. Management of acute clavicle fractures *Orthop. Clinics of N Am.* 2008;39(4):491–505.

10

Long Bone Fractures

Long bone fractures occur in thick cortical bone and, by definition, are medium- to high-energy injuries. They take the longest of any general type of fracture to heal — a minimum of 3 months and often up to 6 months — since the cortical bone is so thick. Since they heal slowly in adults, issues with loss of reduction in a splint or cast are significant. Rigid internal fixation is the usual treatment with IM rods in the lower extremity and plates in the upper extremity (except for uncomplicated humeral shaft fractures).

Secure fixation allows for early ambulation and joint movement. This is very important in adults where above-elbow or above-knee casting is poorly tolerated and leads quickly to joint stiffness. In contrast, long bone fracture treatment in children generally does not require internal fixation; the fractures heal quicker and even prolonged casting above a joint does not lead to permanent stiffness.

Femoral Shaft Fractures

Femoral shaft fractures are all high-energy injuries since the femur is heavily covered with muscle and very strong. These injuries are typically seen in young males during high-risk sporting activities and in MVAs. A small subgroup of older and elderly adults present with pathological fractures after relatively low-energy trauma.

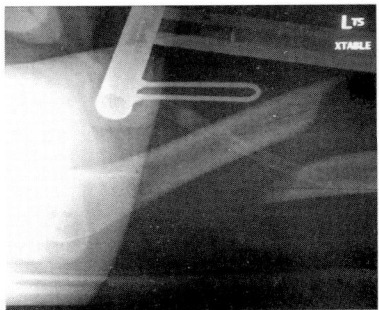

If a patient presents with a femoral shaft fracture after a *low-energy* injury, suspect a pathological fracture.

Figure 10.1 Femoral shaft fracture (Note the typical degree of displacement/shortening.)

Diagnosis is relatively easy clinically and radiographically. Often, the leg is very swollen and shortened. Look for associated injuries in the MSK and elsewhere, as these are high-energy injuries.

These fractures should all be treated with intramedullary fixation, as the fracture and femur are ideally suited for this implant. The procedure is technically demanding, but once completed, with the new titanium locking implants, the patient can usually get out of bed the next day, moving the hip and knee quickly. Weight bearing can progress quickly and, even in noncompliant patients, there are usually few problems with nonunion or malunion. The key is to get the operation done quickly and to do it technically well.

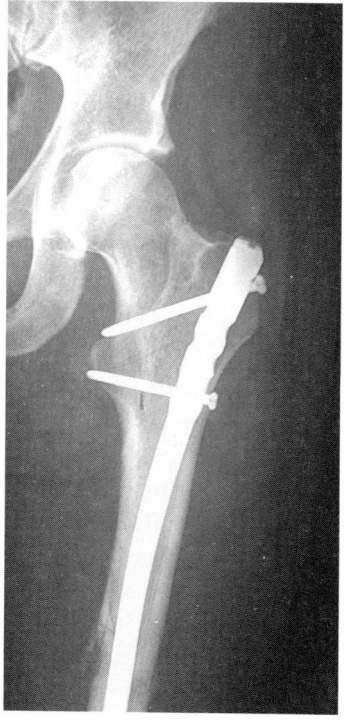

Figure 10.2 Femoral shaft fracture fixed with locked IM nail

The timing of surgery is important: a large body of trauma literature suggests that rigid fixation of long bone fractures (especially femoral shaft) within the first 24 hours after injury significantly reduces the rate of sepsis and chest complications such as ARDS.[1] This is particularly true in the multitrauma patient. Even in the young male with an isolated femoral shaft fracture, early IM nailing of the fracture is associated with a decreased incidence of fat embolism syndrome.[2]

Features of the fat embolism syndrome include the following:

- hypoxia of various degrees
- low-grade fever
- patient can be mildly confused
- subconjuctival petechiae
- low platelets on CBC
- CXR can be normal

- patchy or diffuse infiltrates (ARDS); major differential diagnosis is PTE; most cases mild and self-limiting with supportive care; a few cases end up in the ICU with ARDS

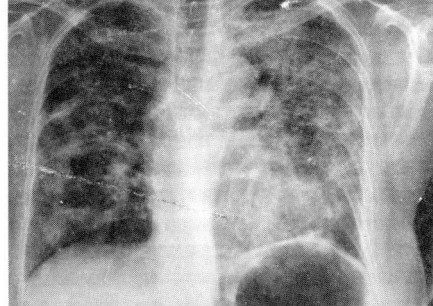

Figure 10.3 ARDS on CXR

For these reasons, IM nailing of all femoral fractures within the first 24 hours, especially in young men, is critical.

Tibial Shaft Fractures

Tibial shaft fractures are quite common and are seen in a variety of ages and injury settings. Although the tibial shaft is strong, the bone lacks soft tissue coverage and is subcutaneous anteriorly; therefore, it is subject to fractures from direct blows (as well as the usually twisting injuries), and many of these fractures can be open. The lack of soft tissue coverage affects the blood supply, so these fractures can be very slow to heal and are more prone to wound breakdown and infection if the fracture was open.

Two general presentations are seen: (a) low-energy, twisting injuries and (b) higher-energy, direct blows to the tibia.

LOW ENERGY: TWISTING

Isolated, low-energy twisting injuries include boot-top skiing fractures and twisting falls down steps in older adults. For some reason, they are common in alcoholics and present late, the next day, to the emergency department.

Usually, circulation is good and swelling is not significant. Watch the skin over the apex of the deformity in older patients, as it can be quite thin and at risk of breakdown. Realign and splint the extremity. Definitive IM nailing should be done within 72 hours.

HIGH ENERGY: DIRECT BLOW

These tibial shaft fractures occur in high-energy situations, mostly in young patients. This is the classic motorcycle accident fracture (open tibial shaft fracture), but it can be seen with motor vehicle and all-terrain vehicle accidents, as well as industrial accidents.

Because of poor anterior soft tissue coverage, many of these fractures are open injuries. In addition, if the fracture is not open, the high-energy nature of the injury can produce significant soft tissue trauma that can lead to a compartment syndrome situation. Compartment syndromes are more common if the fracture is comminuted, the limb was crushed in some way, or a vascular injury is also present. (See Chapter 3 for a more detailed discussion.)

These fractures definitely need to be fixed earlier than the low-energy group:

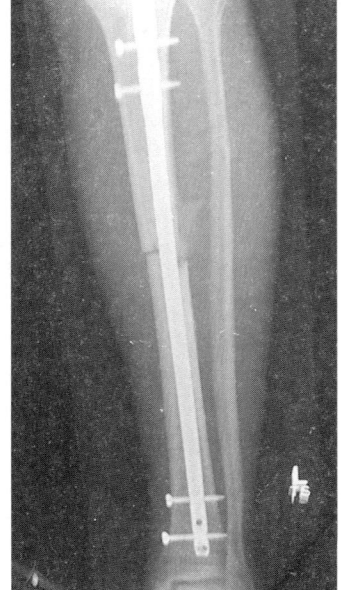

Figure 10.4 Higher-energy tibial shaft fracture, with comminution; IM nail

- if there is an open wound, within 6 hours (debridement and fixation)
- if very swollen and compartment syndrome suspected, within 6 hours for compartment release (fixation at same time or later surgery to follow)
- if closed, but only moderately swollen, within 24 hours for fixation

CHECKLIST OF COMPLICATIONS IN TIBIAL SHAFT FRACTURES

Early: Closed fractures
- compartment syndromes
- DVT

Early: Open fractures
- soft tissue coverage problems
- wound breakdown (Grafts or flaps may be needed.)
- wound infections

Late
- delayed or nonunions
- deep infection/osteomyelitis
- sequelae of nerve or vascular injuries
- chronic swelling/joint stiffness/implant problems

Definitive fixation is still usually an IM nail, but in Grade III open fractures and some compartment syndromes, an external fixation device may be used initially (with later conversion to an IM nail).

The complication rate, especially in the high-energy shaft fracture group, is significant. Most can be traced back to poor soft tissue coverage and blood supply issues inherent to the tibial shaft itself.

For all of these reasons, orthopaedic surgeons have a lot of respect for high-energy, tibial shaft fractures and follow these patients for months or years after the original injury.

Humeral Shaft Fractures

Humeral shaft fractures are not that common but can present after a twisting injury to the upper arm in all age groups. In young people, a lot of force needs to be applied to break the strong humeral shaft. This is the classic "grenade thrower's fracture" or "arm wrestling fracture" seen in muscular men. Most are due to a twisting rotational force, but a few are caused by a direct blow or contusion and are more transverse in character upon X-ray. Older patients with osteoporosis and patients with cancer can present with a pathological humeral shaft fracture after a relatively minor twist to the upper arm.

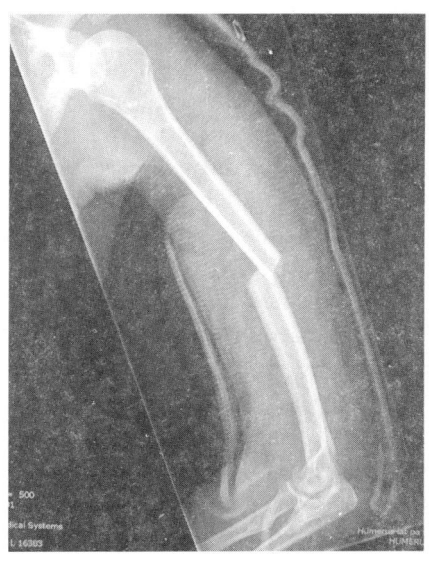

Figure 10.5 Displaced mid-shaft fracture of humerus

Diagnosis is easy clinically and radiographically. Long spiral fractures are more stable than short transverse patterns. Mid-shaft fractures are more stable than distal third fractures.

The radial nerve is at risk in the mid- to distal third of the humerus. Injuries of the radial nerve are not uncommon in the higher-energy fracture type but, fortunately, most deficits are temporary.

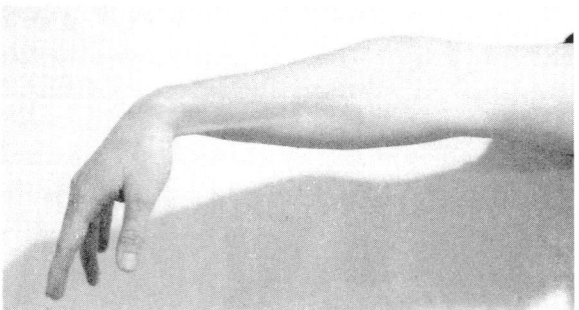

Figure 10.6 Classic wrist drop from radial nerve injury

Uncomplicated humeral shaft fractures are the one exception to the general rule that long bone fractures should be treated with early fixation. Most humeral shaft fractures in the central two-thirds of the shaft can be treated quite nicely with serial splints and then custom orthotics. Specifically, a "sugar tong splint" is applied in the E.R. (anterior/posterior above-elbow half splint with a shoulder immobilizer to splint to the chest for comfort). The patient is seen in 7–10 days, re-X-rayed, and a new sugar tong splint applied as swelling has decreased. The patient is seen every 2 weeks and adjustments are made according to the X-ray.

Gravity assists the fracture in alignment, so these patients should initially sleep in a reclining chair. The hanging cast has been used previously for this gravity-assisted reduction of humeral fractures, but the sugar tong splint is more comfortable for patients. At 6 weeks, the patient is usually ready to be converted to a custom-made upper arm orthotic, which should be worn 23 hours per day for the next 6 weeks.

Healing is usually solid by 3–4 months. Refracture can be a concern in active young patients. The return to sports activities should be put off for 6 months.

Certain humeral shaft fracture patterns (perhaps < 15%) are more unstable or problematic and are not well suited for closed splinting. Their characteristics are as follows:

- short transverse/oblique fractures with marked displacement
- distal fractures at the metaphyseal flare (collapse into varus)
- noncompliant or obese patients (cannot tolerate splint)
- multitrauma patients (need to be mobilized quickly)

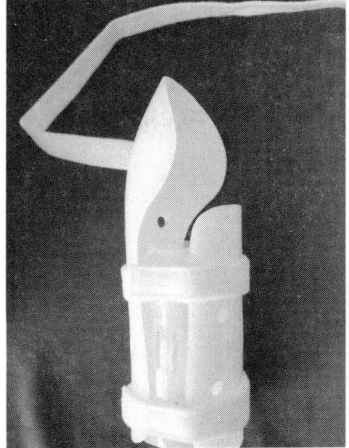
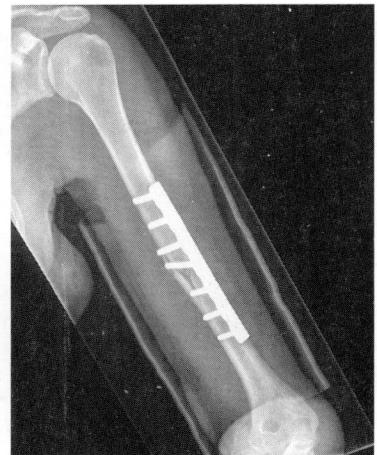

Figure 10.7 Sugar tong orthotic

Figure 10.8 Fixation of humerus shaft fracture (failed splinting)

- persistent malposition despite serial adjustments
  · angulation > 20 degrees; no apposition of fragments
- pathological fractures from cancer

In these cases, the fracture is usually fixated with a large plate and screws. Pathological fractures are generally best treated with IM nails.

Most patients with humeral shaft fractures do well with conservative treatment and heal in 3–4 months. The X-rays do not have to show perfect alignment: AP or lateral malangulation of < 15 degrees is quite acceptable and allows for good function. The major problem encountered is usually shoulder and elbow stiffness. Gentle ROM exercises should be started at the elbow and the shoulder by 2 weeks postinjury. No weights should be used for the first 3 months. However, if a delayed union or malunion is developing, or a failure of conservative treatment is becoming more obvious, surgical treatment should be started earlier rather than later. Stiffness around the shoulder and elbow only worsens with the passage of time.

Forearm Shaft Fractures

The forearm, like the lower leg and the pelvic ring, is a closed two-bone system. It is rare, in an adult, to have a displaced fracture of one bone without a fracture or dislocation of the other bone. The only exception is an isolated, usually mildly displaced fracture of the ulna

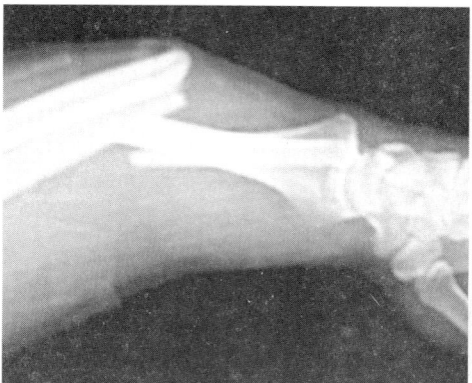

Figure 10.9 Displaced fractures of radius and ulna

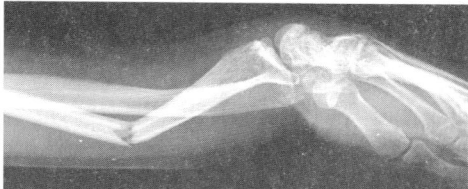

Figure 10.10 Galeazzi fracture/dislocation

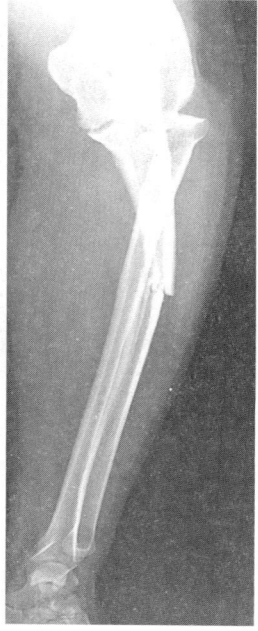

Figure 10.11 Monteggia fracture/dislocation

from a direct blow to the bone ("night stick fracture" < 5% cases). In-direct injuries will follow one of the following three patterns:

- fracture both the radius and ulna (usually mid-shaft and dis-placed); the most common pattern seen (> 90% cases)
- fracture the radius and dislocate the ulna at the wrist (Galeazzi fracture/dislocation); dramatic, but uncommon injury (< 1% cases)
- fracture the ulna and dislocate the radial head at the elbow (Monteggia fracture/dislocation (< 5% cases); can be missed if angulation is mild

Most of these injuries are medium to high energy in nature. A lot of force is necessary to break these strong cortical bones or dislocate these joints.

In the E.R., these injuries should be splinted and checked for pos-sible open wounds (often on the subcutaneous border of the ulna or at the apex of the fracture deformity) and nerve injuries (especially

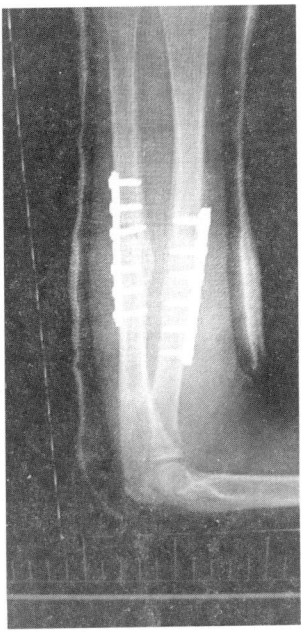

Figure 10.12 ORIF of forearm fractures — must be precise

with fracture/dislocations). Moderate swelling is common, but beware of crush injuries and highly displaced fractures, which can produce a compartment syndrome of the forearm.

Regardless of the pattern, almost all these fractures are unstable, are impossible to reduce by closed means, or will drift in a cast, so ORIF with plates and screws is the rule. Surgery should be done within 24–48 hours unless an open injury or compartment syndrome is present (6 hours). Operative fixation must be precise because the forearm bones must work as a unit and rotate around one another at the wrist and elbow. Malunions are poorly tolerated in the forearm. If the fracture in the bone is reduced and plated anatomically, usually the dislocation reduces itself; formal open reduction of the joint is rarely needed.

Most of these injuries do quite well if they are treated aggressively with precise internal fixation and the soft tissues were not damaged too much from the original injury. Other complications include wrist and elbow stiffness, loss of forearm rotation (usually supination), tendonitis from prominent screws and plates, and residual nerve damage from the original injury.

REFERENCES

1. Behrman SW, Fabian TC, Kudsk KA, et al. Improved outcome with femur fractures: early vs. delayed fixation. *J Trauma*. 1990;30(7):792–8, discussion 797–8. http://dx.doi.org/10.1097/00005373-199007000-00005. Medline:2380996

2. Kosova E, Bergmark B, Piazza G. Fat embolism syndrome: clinician update. Circ. 2015;131:317–20.

11

Elbow Injuries

Elbow injuries are reasonably common and run the spectrum from low- to medium- to high-energy injuries. The high-energy injuries can be very difficult to reconstruct and have a high complication rate. However, even low-energy injuries can produce a stiff elbow, which is the major problem after any injury around the elbow. The elbow should be gently moved, therefore, as soon as safely possible after any elbow injury (7–21 days). If reduction/fixation does not allow this, then it is inadequate.

Heterotopic ossification (HTO) is potentially a problem after any elbow injury, particularly in young muscular patients. This can also produce significant elbow stiffness. Regularly prescribed NSAIDs for the first month after injury have been shown to decrease HTO in some studies and should be considered in high-risk cases.[1]

> The elbow joint is very prone to stiffness after any injury.

Low-Energy Injuries

Radial Head Fractures

These are common in young and middle-aged adults after a fall onto the elbow with a valgus force applied. The elbow is tender and swollen laterally and elbow motion is limited (particularly rotation). X-rays show a radial head fracture, with various amounts of displacement and angulation. We use the "rule of thirds" to determine the need for operative intervention:

- ORIF if > one-third radial head surface; and > 3 mm displacement; or > 30 degrees of valgus angulation

Fortunately, 90% of these fractures are not this displaced and can be treated conservatively:

- removable above-elbow splint < 3 weeks

- early gentle ROM elbow
- early referral to physio-therapy

As mentioned, even these minimally displaced, seemingly trivial, radial head fractures can lead to permanent elbow stiffness, so warn your patients of this possibility and be vigilant with early ROM.

Extra-articular Supracondylar Humerus Fractures

These are uncommon injuries but are seen in the elderly or in patients with severe osteoporo-

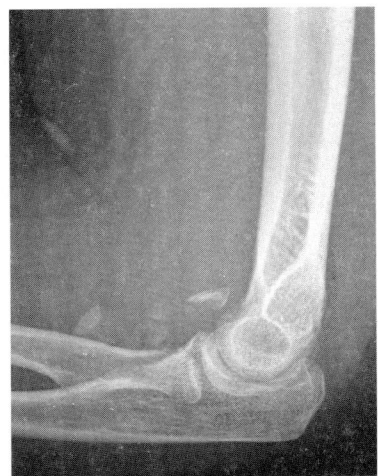

Figure 11.1 Comminuted radial head fracture

sis after a fall on the elbow. The metaphyseal flare of the distal humerus becomes the weak link around the elbow (rather than the radial head or the joint capsule), so the fracture is extra-articular, impacted, and usually into valgus.

Treatment is usually conservative (unless angulation is significant, > 20 degrees, which is unusual):

- above-elbow splinting for 3 weeks
- early ROM + hinged brace or orthotic
- surgery can be difficult due to poor bone quality

Distal Biceps Tendon Ruptures

Distal biceps tendon ruptures are not common, but they are quite dramatic when they do occur, usually in muscular men 30–50 years old (often those who lift weights). Typically, the man is lifting with the elbow extended in an awkward position

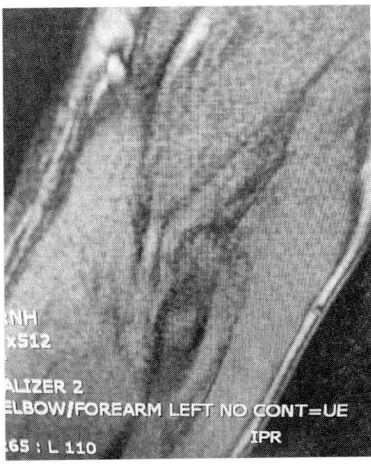

Figure 11.2 MRI of distal biceps tendon tear

when he feels a painful pop or tearing in the elbow. He loses elbow strength and notices a deformity of the biceps muscle (bunching up of the muscle proximally).

Diagnosis is straightforward. Plain X-rays are usually normal. (Elbow arthritis or a bony avulsion from the proximal radius is rare.) An ultrasound can be helpful to determine if the tear is partial or complete.

Treatment should be individualized to each patient. Many patients have a relatively minor biceps deformity and, if they have good early elbow ROM and strength, can be treated with temporary elbow splinting, physiotherapy, and a gradual return to work and sports. Other patients are unhinged by the appearance of the deformity, are quite weak, and want the problem fixed surgically.

Surgery is much easier if done in the first 2 weeks after injury (as the muscle retracts and scars down). The distal biceps tendon must be reanchored to the bicipital tuberosity area with some form of suture anchor, deep in the elbow, and is a tricky operation. Patients must be careful for up to 3 months after surgery to prevent rerupture. In addition, due to the nature of the soft tissue dissection, scarring and HTO can occur postoperatively around the elbow with potential permanent loss of elbow motion (particularly forearm supination). This can be more disabling than the loss of power from the original biceps rupture, so patients undergoing surgery should be warned of this complication.

Medium-Energy Injuries

Olecranon Fractures

Olecranon fractures can occur in all age groups from a fall directly onto the point of the flexed elbow.

Diagnosis is straightforward on radiographs. Most fractures with distraction of fragments > 5 mm will need operative fixation. If the fracture is minimally displaced, ask the patient to actively extend the elbow against gravity: if they are able to, then the extensor mechanism is intact and surgery is not necessary; if they cannot, then even < 5 mm of distraction has disrupted the extensor mechanism and surgery is required. Surgery involves olecranon wiring (or plating) and early elbow ROM (by 3 weeks). Patients usually do well, but many require removal of the subcutaneous wires once the fracture is healed since there is very little soft tissue coverage.

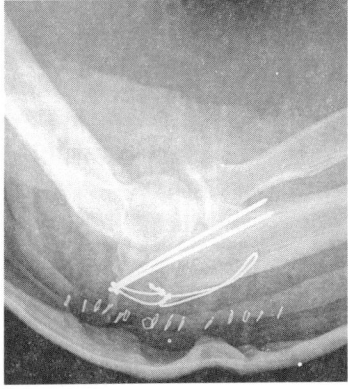 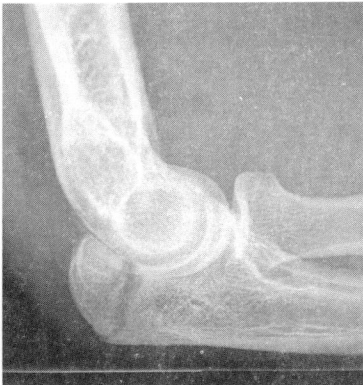

Figure 11.3 Olecranon fracture pre- and post-fixation

Elbow Dislocations

The elbow is not a joint that is commonly dislocated, but young adults and middle-aged adults, particularly if they have some measure of lax joints in general, can be injured in this way. The elbow looks dramatically deformed. X-rays in two planes confirm the diagnosis. The elbow dislocates posteriorly/laterally more often than posterior/medially.

Look for small avulsion fractures from the medial humeral epicondyle, radial head, or coronoid process. Most of these can

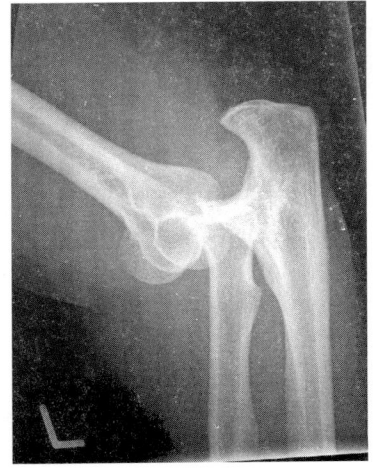

Figure 11.4 Posterior elbow dislocation

be gently reduced in the E.R. under sedation. If fractures are large, then this is more than a simple dislocation and reduction should be done in the O.R. by an orthopaedic surgeon. Ligament repair or fracture fixation may be required in these cases to get the elbow reduced and stable.

Careful follow-up is needed to assess stability and timing of physiotherapy. (All patients should be moving the elbow within 2–3 weeks.) Elbow stiffness and HTO can be complications.

High-Energy Injuries

Intra-articular Distal Humerus Fractures

These are high-energy, very serious fractures of the axial load or shear type seen in young and middle-aged adults after falls from significant heights, industrial accidents, or MVAs. These fractures can be open (since the bones are quite subcutaneous), and nerve injury is possible due to their proximity crossing the elbow.

Operative fixation is very technically demanding. Most of these elbows will have some residual disability and an increased risk of post-traumatic elbow osteoarthritis. Start ROM postoperatively and consider NSAIDs early.

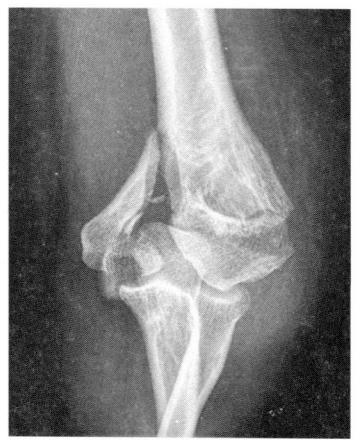

Figure 11.5 High-energy distal humerus fracture

Elbow Dislocations with Significant Associated Fractures

THE UNHAPPY TRIAD: RADIAL HEAD, CORONOID PROCESS, AND OLECRANON

These high-energy, fortunately rare, elbow injuries on first appearance look like simple elbow dislocations/fractures. However, the force involved is higher and on closer inspection of the plain X-rays, more significant fractures are identified in structures that normally stabilize the elbow (i.e., the radial head, the olecranon, the coronoid process, or the distal humerus). These can be tricky to diagnose. These are very serious injuries and should not be underestimated because the fragments

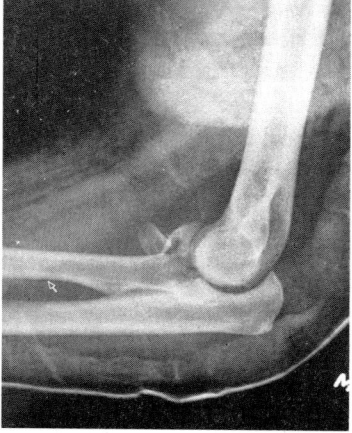

Figure 11.6 High-energy elbow injury (radial head, coronoid process and elbow subluxation)

are small on initial X-rays. If in doubt about whether a fragment is significant, order a CT of the elbow and involve an orthopaedic surgeon early.

At surgery, these injuries are very technically demanding to repair. Fractures and ligaments need to be repaired in a stepwise order until the elbow is stable.

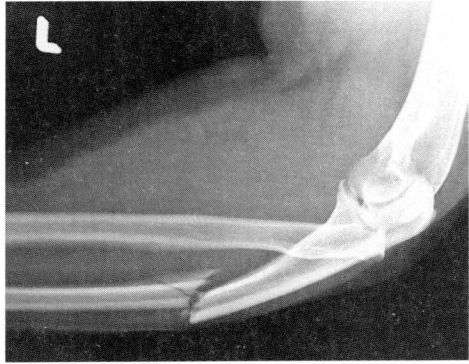

Figure 11.7 Monteggia fracture/dislocation of left elbow (Radial head is subluxed posteriorly.)

Postoperatively, the elbow will have some residual disability, including recurrent instability or stiffness, possible HTO, and post-traumatic osteoarthritis.

MONTEGGIA TYPE

These elbow fracture/dislocations were described previously in the forearm section in Chapter 10. Although they are medium- to high-energy injuries, they are easier to fixate because the ulna fracture is easy to plate and the radial head readily relocates. These injuries do much better than the more complex unhappy triad elbow dislocations.

In summary, all injuries around the elbow need to be diagnosed and treated early so the elbow is stable and can be moved early to minimize ongoing stiffness.

Elbow stiffness is the number one enemy when dealing with elbow injuries!

REFERENCE

1. Hildebrand KA, Patterson SD, King GJW. Acute elbow dislocations: simple and complex. *Orthop Clin North Am.* 1999;30(1):63–79. http://dx.doi.org/10.1016/S0030-5898(05)70061-4. Medline:9882725

12

Foot

Foot injuries, taken as a group, are quite common when the forefoot is included. The severity of the injury and complexity of the fracture usually increases as one moves from the forefoot to the mid-foot to the hind-foot. By definition, the *forefoot* extends from the toes distally to the metatarsal bases; the *mid-foot* from the metatarsal/cuneiform joint distally to the talonavicular and calcaneal–cuboid joint proximally; and the *hind-foot* includes the talus and calcaneus bones and the subtalar and ankle joints.

Forefoot Injuries

Forefoot injuries include the metatarsals (MT) and the toe phalanges. They occur in all age groups, usually from falling objects and crush injuries. The exception to this would be the avulsion fracture at the base of the fifth metatarsal, which occurs from a twisting injury to the foot. In general, the first and fifth toes and metatarsals are the most important since they are the border toes: deformities look worse cosmetically, and weight bearing goes through the great toe to a large degree. Much more displacement and angulation can be tolerated for D2–D4 metatarsal and phalangeal fractures than D1 and D5 toes and metatarsals.

Swelling can be significant for any crush injury, so splint and elevate the foot and keep the patient non-weight bearing initially; then decide if all the joints are reduced and the fracture patterns are stable. If so, keep them non-weight bearing for 2–4 weeks and then begin gradual weight bearing in an air boot for the next 4–8 weeks. Complete healing can still take 3 months.

Fifth metatarsal fractures at the base in metaphyseal bone are quite common and will heal without surgery (but may take 2–3 months in an air boot). They are different from the true Jones fracture of the proximal one-third shaft area of the fifth metatarsal, which has a high nonunion rate.

If there are dislocations or unstable fracture patterns, intervention is necessary. Closed reduction and splinting (or buddy taping) is indicated for isolated single MTP or IP joint toe dislocations with no associated large fractures.

SURGICAL INDICATIONS FOR FOREFOOT INJURIES

Surgery is indicated for the following:

- irreducible single toe dislocations
- multiple toe dislocations or fracture/dislocations
- displaced intra-articular IP, MTP, or MT/cuneiform fractures
- displaced or angulated fractures of first or fifth MT shaft, or great toe proximal phalanx
- displaced fractures of the fifth MT proximal one-third shaft area (Jones fracture)

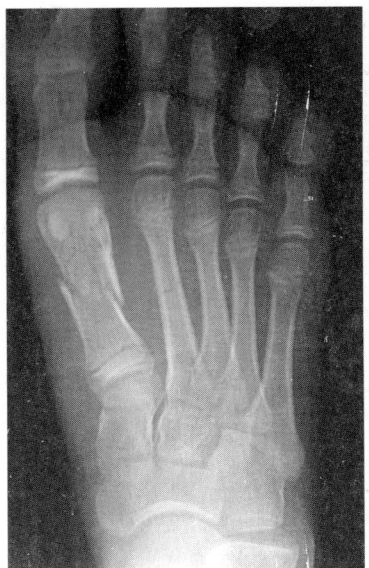

Figure 12.1 Displaced first metatarsal fracture

Significant displacement usually means less than 50% of bone apposition or malangulation of 20 degrees or more.

Fixation techniques include removable K-wires and/or mini-plates/screws. Joints must be reduced and congruent, and the overall alignment of the MT rays should be parallel.

Mid-foot Injuries

Mid-foot injuries are not common, but they are important and are seen in moderate- to high-energy twisting injuries. The classic mechanism is twisting the foot in a stirrup while falling off a horse, which produces the so-called Lis Franc injury, described during one of the Napoleonic wars. This is a mid-foot fracture/dislocation through the bases of the metatarsals, which can be isolated to the first and sec-

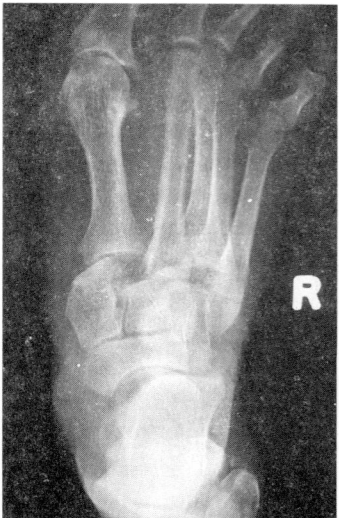

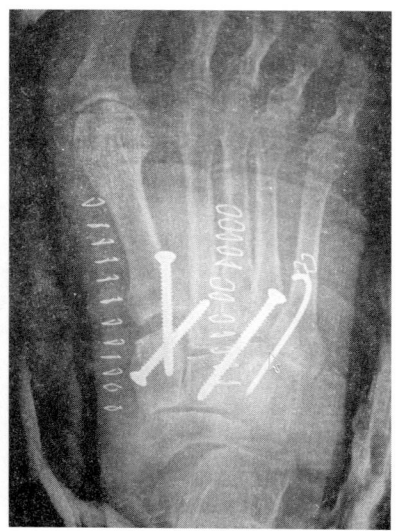

Figure 12.2 Lis Franc injury (Note the
lateral drift of the MT bases.)

Figure 12.3 ORIF of Lis Franc (Note normal
parallel columns have been restored.)

ond metatarsal or involve all five. Today, we see this injury more commonly after motorcycle or all-terrain vehicle accidents.

Clinically, the mid-foot is quite swollen. Diagnosis can be tricky on X-rays for some of the more subtle fractures: X-ray the uninjured foot if in doubt. Study the plain X-rays carefully — AP, lateral, and oblique views — to ensure the metatarsal columns line up in parallel with the mid-foot bones (base of first MT with lateral border of medial cuneiform; medial border of fourth MT with medial border of cuboid bone). If the columns do not line up, then the whole ligamentous integrity of the mid-foot joint is damaged and the metatarsals will drift laterally. This will only worsen with time and weight bearing. Look, in particular, at the base of the second metatarsal, for it is the keystone of stability for the mid-foot.

These are unstable injuries and early operative fixation is required for any displaced Lis Franc fracture/dislocation. A few will be non-displaced and can be treated conservatively, but the majority will be displaced.

A full 3 months is needed for healing and the foot will be stiff for months afterward. Late osteoarthritis can develop in the affected joints. If displaced initially, these are significant injuries.

Other, less common mid-foot injuries include isolated navicular or cuboid bone fractures (so called "Nutcracker fractures" — related to their mechanism of injury). Most of these are minimally displaced and can be treated conservatively. Localized ORIF is needed for displaced fractures.

Hind-foot Injuries

Hind-foot injuries are usually moderate- to high-energy fractures in young or middle-aged adults (rare in the elderly and children).

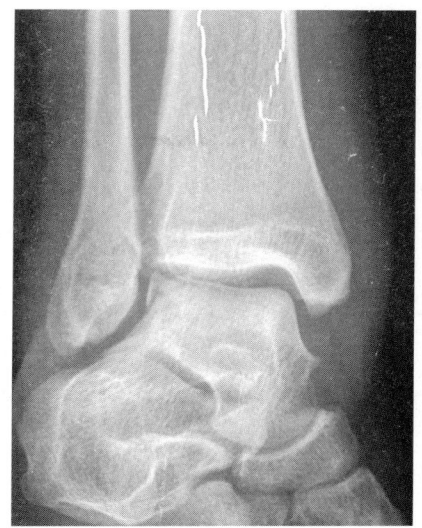

Figure 12.4 Anterior lateral talar dome fracture

They can involve the talus or the calcaneus, and their respective joints.

Talar Injuries

TALAR DOME OSTEOCHONDRAL IMPACTION FRACTURES

These are not common but can cause chronic disability. They are typically seen in young patients after a bad landing during jumping sports. The talar dome is impacted into the distal tibia. The ankle is swollen and the patient cannot weight bear.

X-rays show no ankle fracture, but a small impaction fracture of the anterior lateral or anterior medial corner of the talar dome. Some of these cases are actually "acute on chronic OCD" (osteochondritis dissecans) of the talar dome and have a typically larger and antero-medial talar dome defect. A CT scan is helpful in defining the lesion.

Treatment is conservative with splinting, early motion, and gradual weight bearing. If the fragment is large (> 1 cm) or displaced, arthroscopic or open debridement/drilling may be indicated, so referral to an orthopaedic surgeon is reasonable for larger lesions.

TALAR NECK FRACTURES

Talar neck fractures are uncommon, high-energy injuries that are very important due to their high complication rate if displaced ini-

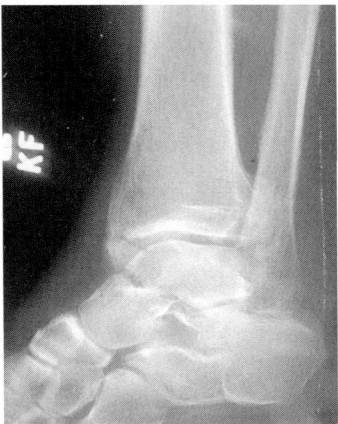

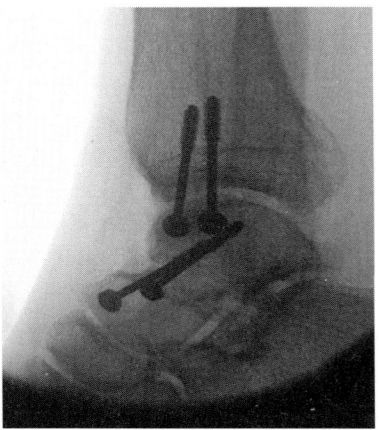

Figure 12.5 Displaced Hawkins II talar neck fracture (plus associated medial malleolus fracture)

Figure 12.6 ORIF of talar neck fracture with screws (in talar neck and medial malleolus)

tially. The talus is one of the bones in the body, along with the hip and scaphoid, that has a retrograde blood supply and is at risk for AVN and nonunion after displaced neck fractures. These injuries are seen after high-energy falls from heights and vehicular accidents where the dorsiflexed foot is loaded violently — the classic pilot plane crash or "aviator's astragalus" injury.

Plain X-rays of the foot make the diagnosis. Injuries are classified according to the amount of talar neck displacement, from nondisplaced to right out the back of the foot and ankle joints (Hawkins I–IV).[1] Only Hawkins I nondisplaced fractures can be treated conservatively, with splinting and gradual progression to weight bearing over 2–3 months. Meticulous ORIF is needed for Types II–IV fractures (ideally within 24 hours because of AVN issues).

Even with early, stable, open reduction of talar neck fractures, the complication rate is high, particularly with the higher-grade injuries. These fractures heal very slowly and AVN and nonunion are common. The talar dome can collapse and early ankle joint osteoarthritis is the inevitable result. Reconstructive procedures can be difficult because of bone loss. Therefore, these patients need to be kept in protective weight bearing for months and followed by an orthopaedic surgeon for at least 2 years to determine the initial healing/outcome. They are very serious injuries.

SUBTALAR DISLOCATIONS (BASKETBALL FOOT)

This injury is very uncommon but is mentioned for completeness. Typically, a tall young man with flexible joints is playing basketball, or another jumping sport, and lands awkwardly on the outside edge of his inverted foot, resulting in a dislocation of the subtalar and mid-foot joint or acute clubfoot deformity. The clinical appearance is very dramatic and X-rays confirm the diagnosis.

Reduction can be performed in the E.R. or O.R. Usually, the injury is stable once reduced and these injuries do well.

Calcaneal Fractures

Calcaneal fractures are serious medium- to high-energy injuries seen most commonly in high-risk-taking men: roofers, snowboarders, climbers, partygoers who jump off balconies. These are not the easiest patients to look after; many are WCB cases, and compliance is often a problem with treatment.

The foot injury is obvious, as it is extremely painful and swollen. Do not forget to look for other injuries from a fall, particularly lumbar spine compression fractures. Soft tissue swelling can be impressive and fracture blisters around the heel are common. These injuries need to be placed in a loose, removable splint and the foot kept elevated for the first 72 hours.

Plain X-rays of the foot and calcaneus should be studied for where the fracture lines extend (into the subtalar joint), loss of the normal height of the calcaneus (Bohler's angle), and amount of widening of the calcaneus on AP views.

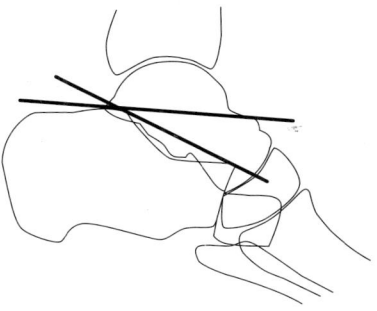

Figure 12.7 Bohler's angle

A CT scan is usually ordered to determine the precise fracture pattern and status of the joints around the calcaneus. Imaging of the foot and calcaneus will determine the general type of calcaneal fracture: (a) joint depression intra-articular type or (b) extra-articular calcaneal tuberosity type.

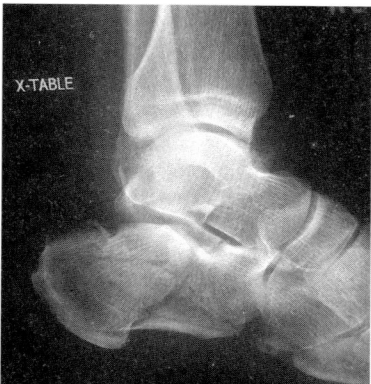

Figure 12.8 Intra-articular calcaneal fracture (Bohler's angle is flat.)

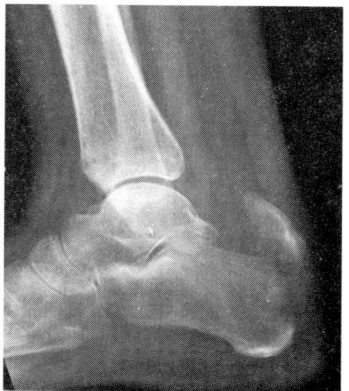

Figure 12.9 Avulsion fracture of calcaneal tuberosity in weak bone

INTRA-ARTICULAR JOINT DEPRESSION FRACTURES

Most calcaneal fractures (80%) will extend into the subtalar joint and will have some flattening of the Bohler's angle. The heel will also widen as it loses height. Mild amounts of displacement can be tolerated, but if Bohler's angle approaches 0 degrees and the subtalar joint shows a step of more than 3–5 mm on CT, then surgery should be considered.

Indications for surgery vary widely and depend on the age of the patient, the quality of the bone, whether the patient smokes, and the projected compliance for treatment. In most centres, there is one orthopaedic surgeon in the group who does all these fixations since the surgery is technically demanding and complications are common (particularly skin breakdown over the incision and infection). Good reviews for operative versus nonoperative treatment of calcaneal fractures exist.[2]

Disability is common regardless of treatment. These patients will be off work for 3–6 months. They have trouble walking on uneven surfaces or on roofs; the heel is wide, producing footwear problems, and many have chronic pain and can develop subtalar joint osteoarthritis. A subsequent subtalar joint fusion may be needed in some of these patients. The foot is never really the same after a significant intra-articular calcaneal fracture.

EXTRA-ARTICULAR CALCANEAL TUBEROSITY FRACTURES

These fractures are in the minority of calcaneal fractures. They are lower-energy injuries, are not generally displaced much, and do not involve the subtalar joint.

Generally, they are treated nonoperatively, with splinting and then graduated protective weight bearing for 2–3 months. Occasionally, in poor bone, part of the calcaneal tuberosity is pulled proximally by the Achilles tendon insertion: these should be repaired surgically.

REFERENCES

1. Hawkins LG. Fractures of the neck of the talus. [Hawkins talar neck classification.]. *J Bone Joint Surg Am.* 1970;52(5):991–1002. Medline:5479485

2. Brauer CA, Manns BJ, Ko M, et al. An economic evaluation of operative compared with nonoperative management of displaced intra-articular calcaneal fractures. *J Bone Joint Surg Am.* 2005;87(12):2741–9. http://dx.doi.org/10.2106/JBJS.E.00166. Medline:16322625

13

Pelvis

Pelvic fractures are not particularly common, and most that one encounters are in elderly patients with stable, low-energy injuries. Broadly speaking, pelvic fractures can be classified into two main groups: (a) low-energy, stable pelvic fractures (> 90% seen) and (b) high-energy, potentially unstable pelvic fractures (< 10%).

Low-Energy Fractures

Low-energy fractures occurring in elderly patients after a ground-level fall are the most common pattern seen in community practice. Often, they present as a possible broken-hip patient. X-rays show no hip fracture and often a subtle inferior pubic ramus fracture. Sometimes the superior pubic ramus is also fractured. These are lateral compression fractures, so often the sacrum has an im-

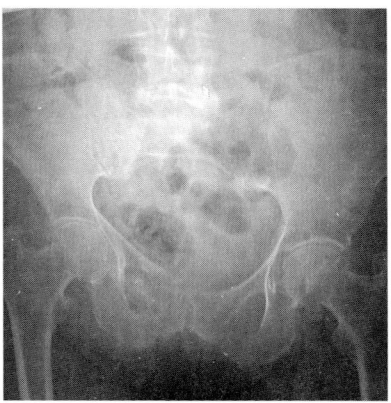

Figure 13.1 Stable right-sided pubic rami fractures in the elderly

pacted fracture on the same side and these patients may experience back as well as groin pain.

These are stable fractures and patients can be ambulated with a walker as soon as they are able. LMW heparin is advisable until they are ambulating normally. Healing takes 3 months radiographically.

High-Energy Fractures

These are fortunately rare in a community hospital setting but commonly seen in major hospitals dealing with multiple trauma cases.

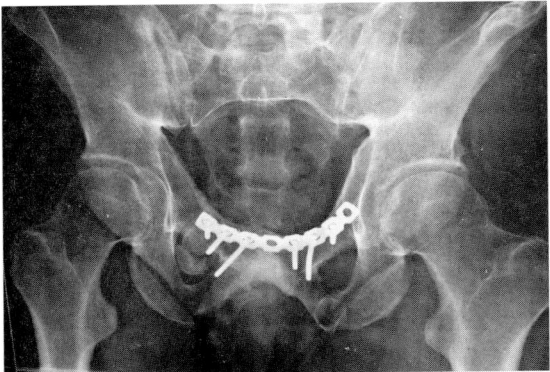

Figure 13.2 Anterior plating for an unstable, open book pelvic fracture

They occur predominantly in young people after major MVAs, riding accidents with horses, and industrial accidents. The bones and ligaments of the pelvis are very strong, so great force is required to produce an unstable pelvic fracture.

The major predictor of whether the pelvic injury is stable or unstable is whether the posterior structures have been disrupted (sacrum, SI joints, or iliac bones). All the weight-bearing forces go through the posterior pelvic ring.

Unstable pelvic fractures are classified into three types, according to Tile[1]: (a) lateral compression, (b) open book, and (c) vertical shear (Malgagne injury).

LATERAL COMPRESSION

- anterior and posterior injury always present
- same or contralateral side of pelvis
- some fractures stable if sacral fracture is impacted

OPEN BOOK

- common injury in horse riding accidents
- unstable if > 2 cm widening of pubic symphysis (SI joints injured)

VERTICAL SHEAR (MALGAGNE INJURY)

- highest-energy injury; always unstable
- high incidence of vascular, urethral injury

CHECKLIST OF SOFT TISSUE INJURIES ACCOMPANYING PELVIC FRACTURE

Venous bleeding
- from the posterior pelvic vessels; can be life threatening
- Military anti-shock trousers (MAST) and an external pelvic fixator may be needed to stabilize the bleeding.

Urethral injuries
- particularly in males
- Check for blood at the urethral meatus and a high-riding prostate *before* inserting Foley catheter.

Nerve injuries
- sacral plexus or branch of sciatic nerve
- can cause permanent deficits (usually a foot drop)

Gastrointestinal (GI) or Genitourinary (GU) visceral damage
- Transfer to a Level I trauma care facility as soon as possible; care will be multidisciplinary.

All of these high-energy pelvic fractures are very serious. Soft tissue injuries are common from the high energy involved in producing the pelvic fracture displacement.

A pelvic ring external fixator is often applied when the patient first goes to the O.R. for venous bleeding control, at the time of laparotomy, or with other lifesaving procedures. This should also ideally be done at the trauma centre and not at the community hospital. These are

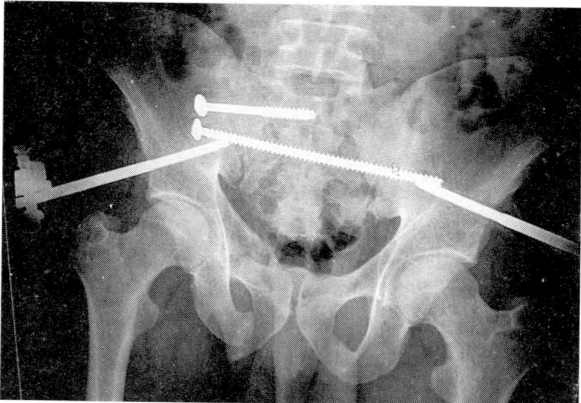

Figure 13.3 ORIF of unstable posterior pelvic fracture complex

really sick patients; for a multitude of reasons, the sooner they are transferred to the trauma centre, the better.

From a bone stability viewpoint, any unstable posterior pelvic injury needs to be stabilized definitely once the patient is stable (usually > 48 hours after the injury). These are large, technically demanding operations and are generally only performed by orthopaedic traumatologists at Level I centres.

There is a high disability rate after a major pelvic fracture. Most patients will take at least 1 year to recover. Problems with chronic pain and nerve impairment (e.g., leg, bladder, sexual function) can be very disabling.

REFERENCE

1. Tile M. Acute pelvic fractures: I. causation and classification. *J Am Acad Orthop Surg.* 1996;4(3):143–51. Medline:10795049

14

Thoracolumbar Spinal Fractures

Spinal fractures will be discussed briefly. As mentioned previously, cervical spine injuries and disorders are beyond the scope of this text.

Thoracolumbar (T/L) spinal fractures do present to community hospitals with isolated injuries and are not automatically sent to tertiary care centres, as is usually the case with C-spine injuries. Fortunately, most of the injuries will be low- to medium-energy fractures in neurologically intact patients with relatively stable fracture patterns.

The key to treating spinal fractures is determining stability of the fracture pattern. Consider the following factors:

- low- versus high-energy injury
- normal versus pathological bone (tumour or infection = unstable)
- associated neural deficit = unstable
- mechanism of injury (becoming increasingly unstable) = flexion → burst → distraction/extension → fracture/dislocation
- number of spinal columns (Denis)[1] involved: two or more = unstable

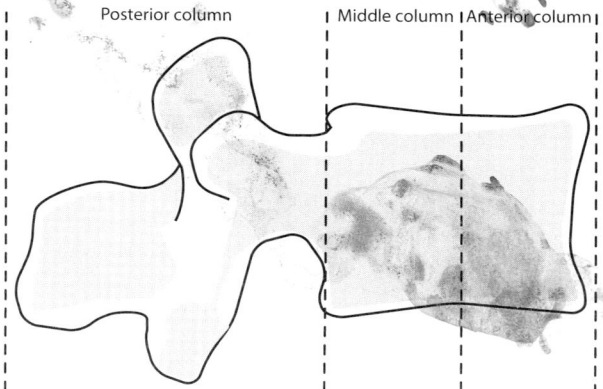

Figure 14.1 Denis three-column spinal fracture classification

Stable Spinal Fractures

Fortunately, in community practice, 90% of the T/L fractures seen are stable, using the criteria previously outlined. They fall into two groups: (a) osteoporotic compression fractures and (b) stable anterior wedge (flexion) fractures.

OSTEOPOROTIC COMPRESSION FRACTURES

These are very common. A frail elderly patient (often female) presents with increasing back pain after a trivial fall, or no fall at all. Clinically, the patient has tenderness in the T/L spine and mild kyphosis.

Plain X-rays show diffuse osteopenia, generalized mild spinal degenerative changes, and one (or more) anterior wedge compression fractures. The appearance is classic, but in this age group, pathological fractures such as infection or tumour (spinal mets or myeloma) should be ruled out. Baseline blood work, CXR, and a CT scan of the affected spinal area are usually prudent. An MRI is not usually needed.

Although the natural history of these fractures is good, many patients will have to be admitted to hospital for pain control. Bedrest is kept to a minimum and they are slowly ambulated with assistance. A back brace may be helpful in some patients (if they can tolerate the inconvenience of wearing it) to ambulate them more quickly. The fracture(s) will take up to 3 months to heal.

These fractures can recur at contiguous spinal levels over many years, giving the spine a kyphotic (Dowager's hump) appearance. Long-term osteoporosis treatment should be started and bone densitometry follow-up arranged in this high-risk group.

STABLE ANTERIOR WEDGE (FLEXION) FRACTURES

These fractures are seen in younger, higher-risk-taking individuals. The thoracolumbar (T10–L2) level is at risk when the spine is subject to a hard landing on the feet. We see these medium-energy injuries in snowboarders, skydivers, vehicular accidents, and falls from heights. Usually, patients can walk and are neurologically intact. They often present to the E.R. one or two days after the injury.

Plain X-rays show an isolated anterior wedge compression fracture with mild kyphosis (< 15 degrees) and no translation of the spinal segment. The anterior column of Denis is always involved.

Occasionally, the middle column is also involved (a so-called burst fracture) and is potentially unstable. A CT scan should be ordered urgently on all patients with this presentation. If the middle column is

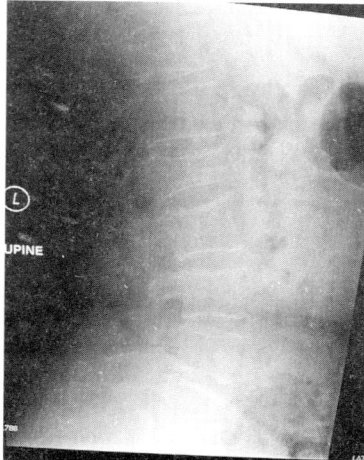

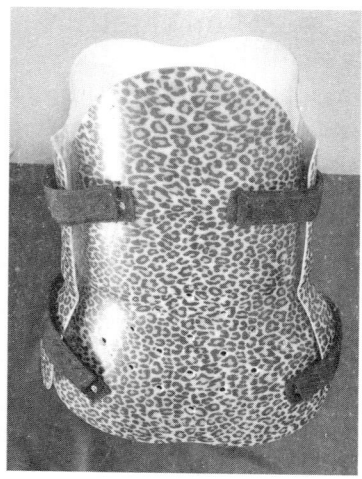

Figure 14.2 Stable L1 wedge fracture

Figure 14.3 TLSO custom brace, clamshell type

involved, then the fracture is potentially unstable. The patient should be admitted and kept on spinal precautions with modified bedrest. Consultation should be obtained on an urgent basis with a spine surgeon who will decide if this particular burst fracture is best treated with a custom thoracolumbar sacral orthosis (TLSO) brace treatment or surgical fixation. Burst fractures have various subtle degrees of instability — from low-energy, relatively stable to high-energy, obviously unstable patterns.

If there is no involvement of the middle column, then the patient may be treated with a back brace as an outpatient and followed for 3 months. The back brace is for comfort and, theoretically, will prevent the kyphosis from progressing.

Unstable Spinal Fractures

Fortunately, these spinal injuries make up less than 10% of the cases seen in a community setting. They occur in young patients after high-energy injuries (vehicular, motorcycle accidents, falls from great heights, and industrial accidents) producing **high-energy burst fractures, extension/distraction injuries,** and **fracture/dislocations of the spine.** They are also seen in older adults with more complicated medical problems (metastatic cancers and diabetes/obesity infections)

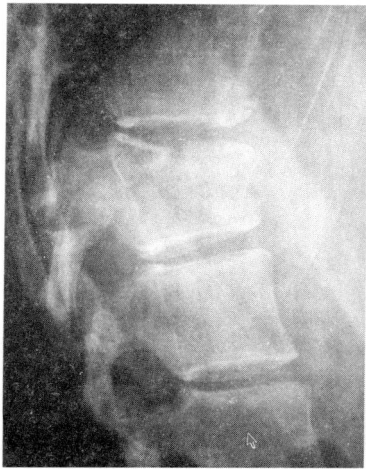

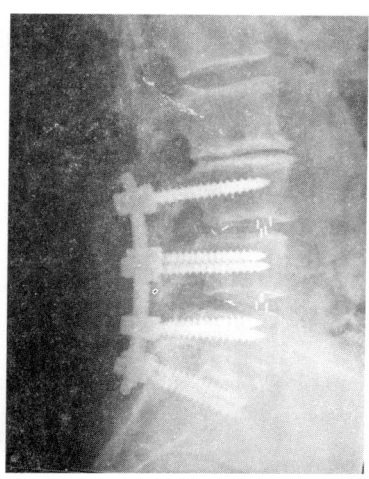

Figure 14.4 Unstable distraction injury through lumbar vertebra and posterior elements

Figure 14.5 ORIF of unstable spinal segment

after relatively minor falls or no injury at all. These patients all have severe pain, cannot walk, and frequently have some neurological deficit.

Plain X-rays typically show misalignment of more than 15 degrees in lateral and/or AP views, possibly with displacement of the spinal segment. In addition, in pathological fractures, a portion of the normal spinal segment seems to be eroded or missing. The overall appearance, even on plain films, looks obviously abnormal and unstable.

These patients should be kept on bedrest with log-rolling precautions and urgently sent for a spinal CT (or an MRI if a nerve deficit is present). A spinal surgeon should be contacted urgently who can decide if IV prednisone loading is warranted and if a spinal cord injury is present. Urgent transfer to a tertiary care centre should then be arranged.

Some form of spinal fixation is performed to stabilize the spinal segment. The type of fixation depends on the mechanism of injury, the status of the neurologic elements, and whether the bone is normal or pathological. This is highly specialized surgery and is normally only done at tertiary care facilities.

REFERENCE

1. Denis F. The three column spine and its significance in the classification of acute thoracolumbar spinal injuries. *Spine*. 1983;8(8):817–31. http://dx.doi.org/10.1097/00007632-198311000-00003. Medline:6670016

15

Pathological Fractures (Hole in Bone)

Pathological fractures have been mentioned to various degrees in previous sections on fractures. However, a few general principles about the workup and management of a "hole in the bone" and pathological fractures will be discussed in this section. This scenario can present in all age groups, but obviously aggressive lesions are much more common in older patients.

Typically, a patient presents with MSK pain that is persistent, nagging, and often worsened by minor trauma. The surprise comes when plain X-rays reveal a hole in the bone or a fracture through obviously weakened bone.

Lesions in bone are best categorized as **nonaggressive versus aggressive** rather than benign versus malignant, as is used in other specialties. This distinction is critical in determining the treatment and ultimate prognosis of the lesion and/or fracture. The process of determining the aggressiveness of the bone lesion is called staging the lesion.

Staging the Lesion: Nonaggressive Versus Aggressive

PLAIN X-RAYS

Close review of plain X-rays forms the cornerstone of tumour staging. Features to look for include the following:

- size of lesion (Smaller is better; large > 10 cm lesions tend to be aggressive.)
- location of lesion (Axial skeletal and more proximal lesions tend to be more aggressive than appendicular distal lesions.)

- margins of the lesion
  · "geographic" (sharp margin) = slowly growing lesion
  · "moth eaten" (gaps in margins) = suggests tumour breakout
  · "permeative" (no clear margins) = rapid, aggressive growth
    = bad
- periosteal reaction (Minimal is good = slow growth; abundant new bone/reaction suggests rapid growth.)
- cortical breakout (Any violation of normal MSK barriers is aggressive tumour behaviour.)
- intrinsic lesion characteristics (clear or homogeneous = good; irregular, speckled calcifications = aggressive)

Examining these features on the initial plain X-rays will allow you to determine generally how aggressive the bone lesion looks. This information will guide you to the next step in staging, and to how urgently you should proceed. Some of these patients with aggressive lesions should be admitted to hospital to expedite the staging of the lesion and future consultations.

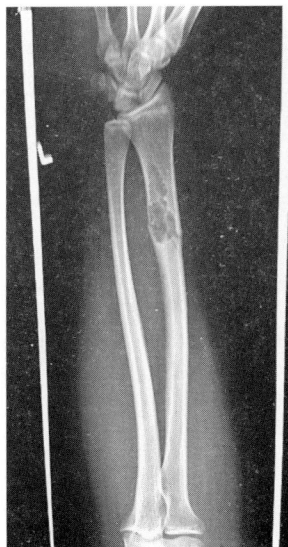

Figure 15.1 Fracture through nonaggressive bone cyst (Note sharp, geographic tumour margins.)

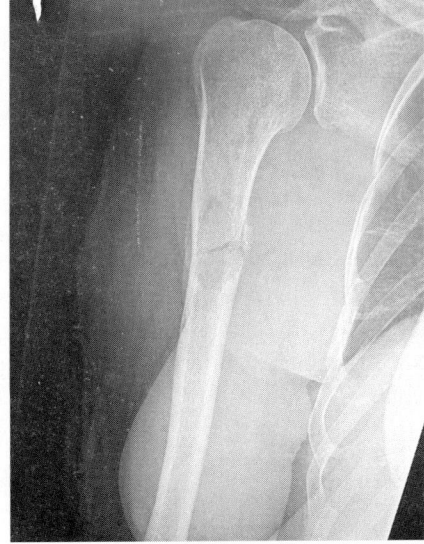

Figure 15.2 Aggressive lesion in humeral shaft from metatstatic tumour (Note indistinct borders, cortical breakthrough and large size of lesion.)

LAB WORKUP

- CBC (Look at red cells, white cells, and platelets.)
- ESR [general indicator of chronic disease or CRP (C-reactive protein)]
- metabolic parameters: electrolytes; creatinine; glucose
- bone metabolism: alkaline phosphatase; calcium; phosphate; serum protein electrophoresis (for myeloma)

SCANS

BONE SCAN AND SKELETAL SURVEY

A bone scan is a somewhat nonspecific but very sensitive test to show increased bone turnover. It will tell you if the lesion is growing quickly, and it will guide you to other areas in the MSK (particularly in the axial skeleton) that have active lesions.

A CXR and plain X-rays of other MSK areas of concern can be ordered, based to some degree on the bone scan findings.

CT SCAN

This is a very good test to look at bony architecture. It can be done very quickly in most community hospitals.

MRI SCAN

The MRI is an excellent test to look at neural elements, particularly in the spine, and to look for soft tissue breakout around the lesion. It is more difficult to arrange than a CT and is not available in all hospitals.

BIOPSY OF LESION

This should be the *very last step* in the staging of the lesion.

Differential Diagnosis

Staging will group the lesions into the two broad categories, nonaggressive and aggressive, and then the patterns seen on the various investigations should provide a diagnosis before tissue biopsy. The following checklist will be useful:

CHECKLIST OF DIFFERENTIAL DIAGNOSIS FOR LESIONS

Nonaggressive, children
- UBC (unicameral bone cyst)
- fibrous cortical defects
- fibrous dysplasia

Nonaggressive, adults
- wedge compression spinal fractures
- fractures through old areas of trauma/indolent infection

Aggressive, children/older teenagers
- leukemia and lymphoma of bone
- osteogenic sarcoma
- Ewings' sarcoma
- infection (osteomyelitis)

Aggressive, adults
- tumours = metastatic much more likely than *primary MSK* (any tissue origin in MSK possible, but rare)
  · chondrosarcoma; GCT; osteogenic sarcoma; muscle and nerve tumours, etc.
  · *multiple myeloma*
  · *metastatic* = > 90% of tumours seen = "benzene ring"
  · *infection:* abscesses and osteomyelitis
  · *metabolic:* renal failure tumours; Ollier's, etc.

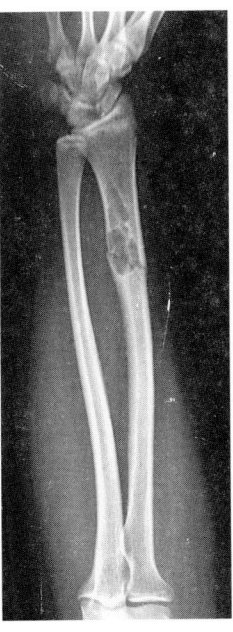

Figure 15.3 Nonaggressive bone lesion in an adolescent boy

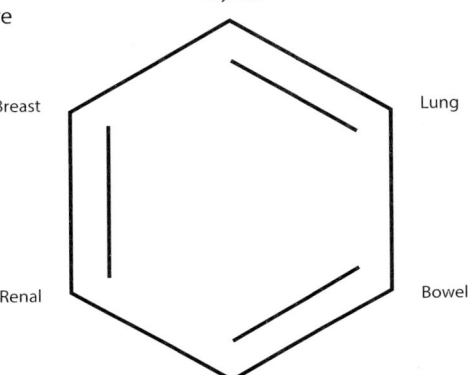

Thyroid

Breast

Lung

Renal

Bowel

Prostate

Figure 15.4 Benzene ring (memory tool): for metastatic tumours that go preferentially to bone

Treatment

Treatment depends on the age of the patient and whether the lesion is nonaggressive or aggressive. Nonaggressive lesions can generally be treated conservatively (with or without a fracture). The fractures will heal in the usual time, and often the cyst will shrink due to the stimulus of the fracture healing. Regular follow-up is prudent.

Aggressive lesions, when the diagnosis is in question, particularly when it may be a primary MSK tumour (such as osteogenic sarcoma), should be referred to an orthopaedic tumour subspecialist for biopsy and definitive surgery. A biopsy in the wrong location could adversely affect specialized limb-sparing surgery in this subgroup of patients. Pre- and post-operative adjuvant therapy is then tailored to the patient and the tumour.

Aggressive lesions obviously related to metastatic cancer, usually associated with a pathological fracture, are often treated by community-based orthopaedic surgeons. Biopsy of the tumour, if needed, is usually obtained from reamings during the IM nailing/fracture fixation procedure.

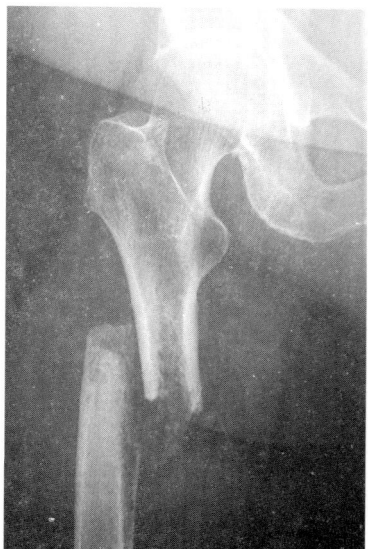

Figure 15.5 Metastatic breast pathological femur fracture (Note indistinct margins and speckled calcification around fracture site.)

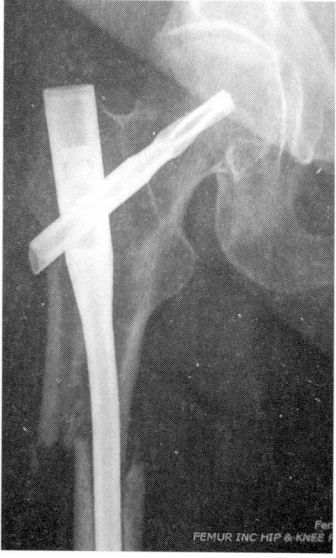

Figure 15.6 IM nail fixation of pathological femur fracture

Although adults presenting with pathological fractures from metastatic lesions have a guarded overall prognosis, they do very well initially with excellent pain relief after fixation of their fractures. IM nail fixation is preferred when possible for long bone fractures because the bone quality is poor. Some tumours can bleed a lot during surgery and patients should be prepared for transfusion. Radiation therapy is often given postoperatively to shrink the tumour mass adjuvantly.

PART THREE

ORTHOPAEDIC TRAUMA IN CHILDREN

16

General Paediatric Principles

Children are not just "small adults" when it comes to fracture care. Generally, the care of children with fractures is very rewarding, since most heal quickly and outcomes are usually good. In addition, the remodelling ability of young bone can also help to improve less-than-perfect reductions. However, some fractures can be quite anxiety provoking to treat, such as elbow fractures, and others must be treated aggressively if they involve the joint or have an unstable fracture pattern. These will be discussed in the following chapters. First, here is an overview of children's fractures.

Healing Times Are Quicker

Fracture healing times depend on blood supply, health of the soft tissues, and quality of the bone, all of which are usually excellent in children. Nonunions are rare in healthy children, but malunions are not uncommon because the bones heal so quickly. Fortunately, most of these malunions are mild, well tolerated, or remodel.

Healing times for specific fractures follow similar trends to those seen in adults but are usually 25–50% shorter, especially in very young children.

Typical healing times:

- phalanges: 3 weeks
- metaphyseal bone (wrists, distal tibia, proximal humerus): 6 weeks
- forearm: 8–12 weeks
- tibial/humeral shaft: 8–12 weeks
- femoral shaft: 12–16 weeks

The fracture must always be evaluated clinically and radiographically to determine if the cast is ready to be removed. Usually, fracture callus is abundant and seen by 2 weeks. Refracture can be a significant problem, particularly in boys, for the first 3 months after cast removal.[1] High-risk sports should be counselled against and a removable splint should be worn until muscle strength and joint motion is normal (generally an additional 4–8 weeks after cast removal).

> Refracture can be a significant problem, particularly in boys, for the first 3 months after cast removal.

Remodelling of Children's Fractures

A unique feature of paediatric bone, remodelling is the process whereby a malunion, with the passage of time and bone growth, will spontaneously correct or improve. The growing bone does this through the elongation of the bone at the growth plate in response to mechanical forces. The fracture does not just round off, as occurs in adults; the distal fragment becomes realigned. This can be quite amazing to see radiographically as you follow the progress of these fractures month by month.

For remodelling to occur, one needs the following:

- open growth plates
- more than 2 years of growth left in the child's bone

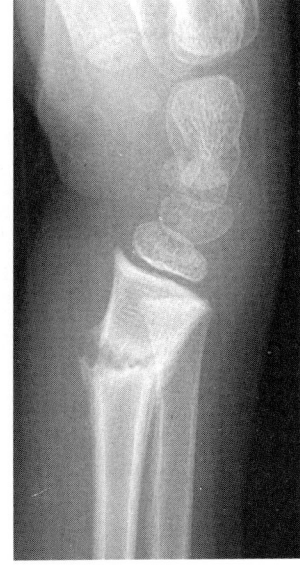

Figure 16.1 Partially healed wrist fracture with dorsal tilting. Will this remodel?

- deformity primarily in the predominant plane of motion of the joint (e.g., dorsal/palmar in wrist; anterior/posterior plane at the ankle)

Fractures usually remodel 10 degrees per year. Malrotation does not remodel.

Determining the number of years of bone growth is an approximate science but follows a few rules. Girls usually stop growing 2 years after the start of their menses and generally have closed growth plates by 14–16 years. Boys usually stop growing later, around 16–18 years. Growth plate closure is related to the stages of puberty and can greatly vary in different cultures and families. There is a wide variation of normal, particularly in boys.

Unique Fracture Patterns in Children

Paediatric bone is very strong, has a good blood supply, and is more elastic than adult bone. In addition to healing quicker than adult bone, it also fails differently in different age groups.

CHECKLIST OF FRACTURE PATTERNS SEEN ONLY IN CHILDREN

Buckle (torus) fractures
- failure of immature metaphyseal bone under compression
- only one cortex buckles
- stable fracture

Greenstick fractures
- seen in long bones
- failure of one cortex in tension/ convex side of the deformity
- stable, but reangulation of fracture common unless fracture "completed" at reduction

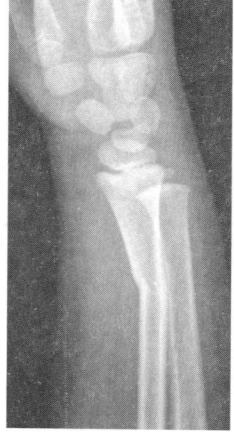

Figure 16.2 Buckle fracture of the distal radius

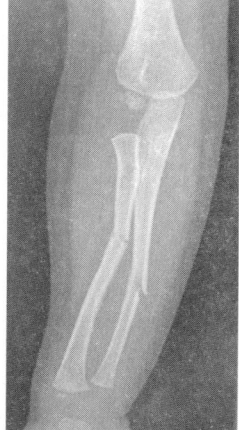

Figure 16.3 Greenstick fracture of ulna; complete fracture of radius

Plastic deformation of long bones
- seen in young children
- cortices of long bone bend but do not break
- need to be reduced to neutral or deformity persists

GROWTH PLATE INJURIES

The Salter-Harris classification system is used universally and should be memorized.

- described by Salter-Harris[2]
- only seen in children, usually aged 6–16, when the growth plate becomes vulnerable to injury

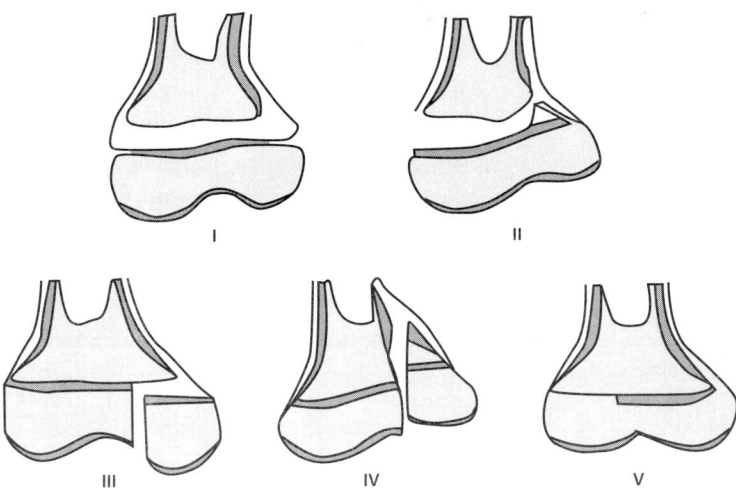

Figure 16.4 Salter-Harris growth plate injury classification system

Salter I

- may be most common Salter fracture
- if no displacement, often diagnosed as a sprain
- seen in wrist and ankle
- tenderness and slight widening of growth plate (or flake of callus seen at edge of physis at 2 weeks)
- immobilize in-situ
- heals quickly

Salter II

- most common seen in practice (when displacement is present)
- extra-articular; easy to reduce; may slip after reduction (K-wires used as adjunct to cast)

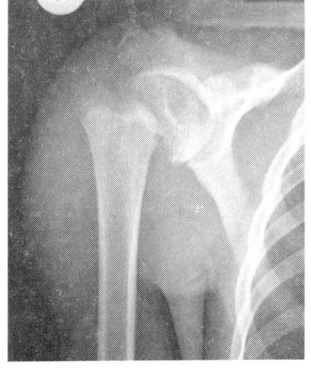

Figure 16.5 Salter II displaced fracture of proximal humerus

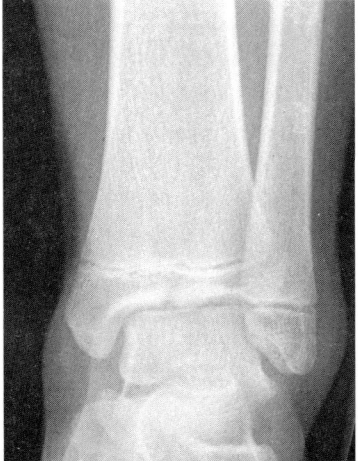

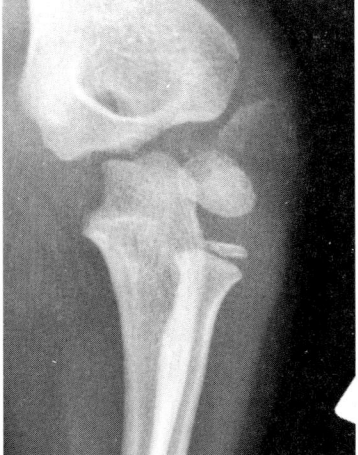

Figure 16.6 Salter III ankle fracture   *Figure 16.7 Salter IV fracture of lateral humeral condyle*

- frequency of sites: distal radius > ankle > proximal humerus > phalanges fingers and toes > distal femur > proximal tibia
- growth arrest can occur, particularly in distal femur; unusual in other anatomic sites

Salter III
- intra-articular
- uncommon overall
- if displaced, one of few indications for open reduction in children
- ankle (Tillaux fracture) and (triplane) ankle fracture
- in older teenagers, physis fuses medially to laterally, so at risk
- ORIF straightforward
- growth arrest uncommon since physis is closing anyway

Salter IV
- intra-articular
- much less common
- if displaced, one of few indications for open reduction in children
- usually seen in varus injuries to the elbow in young children (lateral condyle)
- open reduction is tricky; growth arrest is common (cubitus valgus)

Salter V
- rare, high-energy crush injuries to growth plate
- usually lower limb
- growth arrest after injury may be first clue to diagnosis

Where Is the Weak Link?

We must always ask ourselves, just as with adult fractures, *where is the weak link?* Scaphoid fractures, for example, are rare in children with open growth plates. They are usually seen in older teenagers, usually boys, after age 16. A few generalizations about the weak links in children's bones are outlined in the following checklist.

CHECKLIST OF WEAK LINKS IN CHILDREN'S BONES

Pure dislocations rare in all growing children
- soft tissue and capsule strong
- significant force around a joint usually produces growth plate fracture, metaphyseal fracture, or dislocation with an avulsion fracture (e.g., elbow dislocation with medial epicondyle avulsion)

Open growth plates
- can be a weak link at any age, but especially in the 6- to 15-year age group

Ages 0–5 years
- buckle fractures
- elastic deformation of long bones

Ages 6–11 years
- metaphyseal fractures (wrist, elbow, ankle)
- greenstick forearm
- Salter II injuries

Ages 12–15 years
- apophyseal fractures
- Salter III ankle fractures

Ages 16–18 years
- scaphoid fractures
- long bone fractures

Unique Features of Treatment

Nonunions are rare and displaced intra-articular fractures are uncommon, so the basic treatment of paediatric fractures is closed reduction and casting. Fracture slippage after reduction and malunions are common, so orthopaedists often supplement the closed reduction with smooth percutaneous K-wires that are removed after 3–6 weeks and do not harm the growth plate even if the pin crosses the physis.

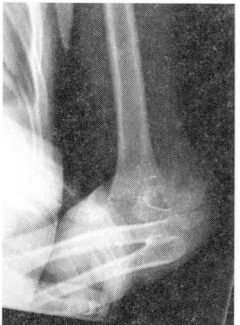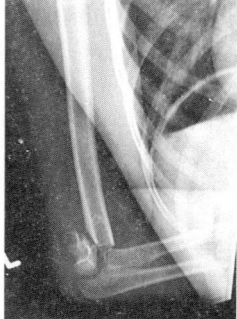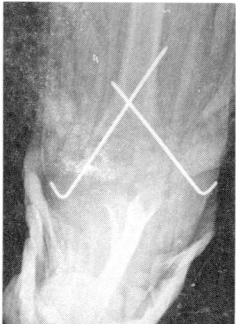

Figure 16.8 Displaced supracondylar humerus fracture pre- and post-fixation with smooth K-wires

Even if formal open reduction of a Salter III or IV fracture is indicated, we often still use limited fixation techniques (such as K-wires or small screws) to limit the potential damage to the growth plate. If plates and screws are used, they are usually small and are often removed once the fracture is healed. The implant does not have to be as sturdy as it is in adult fracture fixation because the fractures heal so much more quickly in children. In addition, children tolerate casts for prolonged periods much better than adults do; this allows us to protect the less robust fixation devices that would fail in adults.

Intramedullary rods are not generally used for femoral or tibial fractures, except in skeletally mature teenagers, again for fear of damaging the growth plate. Instead, a combination of traction and then flexible titanium rods (Nancy nails) is used. These bypass the open growth plates and can also be used in the forearm for very unstable shaft fractures.

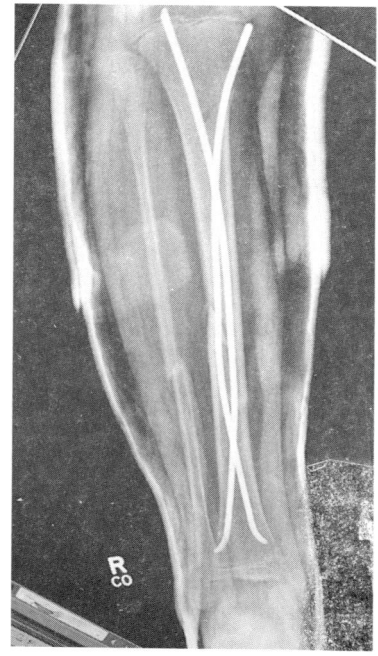

Figure 16.9 Flexible (Nancy) nailing of an unstable tibia fracture

Common Paediatric Fractures

In community practice, the fractures seen most commonly in healthy children involve the wrist/forearm and ankle/distal tibia. These two areas will be discussed in Chapter 17. Elbow fractures, which are not the most common but can be very anxiety provoking and fraught with potential complications, are discussed in Chapter 18. The remaining fractures are then discussed anatomically in Chapter 19.

> The basic treatment of most paediatric fractures is closed reduction and casting.

REFERENCES

1. Rang M, Pring M, Wenger D. Re-fracture rates in forearm fractures *Fractures in Children*. 3rd ed. Lippincott; 2005. p. 135–6.

2. Brown JH, DeLuca SA. Growth plate injuries: Salter-Harris classification. *Am Fam Physician*. 1992;46(4):1180–4. Medline:1414883

17

Most Common Paediatric Fractures

Wrist

Wrist injuries are very common in children, usually resulting from a fall onto the outstretched arm. The exact site of the weak link depends on the age of the child and the amount of energy involved in producing the fracture. The following patterns are common with low- and medium-energy fractures:

- *low energy/young children:* buckle fracture
- *medium energy/young children:* metaphyseal fracture with tilting
- *medium energy/older children:* Salter II fracture with displacement (dorsal > volar)

All these fractures are easy to reduce and generally stable in a below-elbow cast. A primary-care physician who has closed reduction and casting skills could easily manage these fractures.

Sometimes orthopaedic surgeons complement the closed reduction with temporary percutaneous K-wires to prevent reslippage in Salter II wrist fractures. The wires are removed after 3 weeks and a second cast is applied. Generally, these fractures heal within 6 weeks of short-arm casting and most do very well.

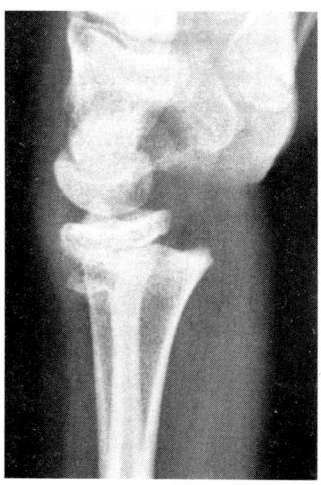

Figure 17.1 Salter II dorsally displaced fracture of distal radius

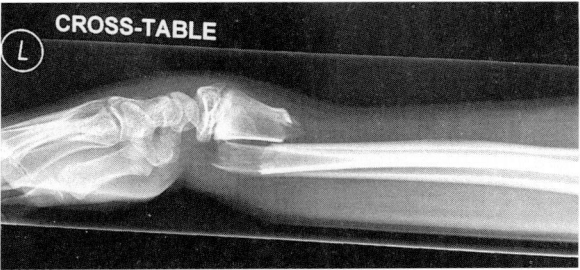

Figure 17.2 Slipper fracture (completely displaced fracture of distal radius)

HIGH ENERGY/OLDER CHILDREN

An important high-energy fracture seen in older children is a completely displaced distal shaft fracture (the "slipper fracture"[1]). These fractures take a lot of force to produce and are tricky to reduce. They should never be reduced under anything but a general anaesthetic and, even then, they are problematic. It is difficult to get the radial fragments hooked on, and the surgeon risks dislocating his own thumbs while attempting to obtain this reduction! Anything less than 50% apposition will probably slip, so one must be prepared to open these fractures and plate or pin them, especially in older children. For all these reasons, these slipper fractures should be referred directly to orthopaedic surgeons.

SCAPHOID FRACTURES

- medium-energy wrist injuries
- rare in children, except older teenagers; usually boys older than 16 years
- below-elbow thumb spica cast for 8–12 weeks
- compliance and refracture can be a problem

Forearm

Forearm fractures are very common and often look dramatic in the emergency department due to the angulation, especially greenstick fractures, but most do very well. There is a continuum of severity, again dependent on the amount of energy necessary to produce the fracture:

- *low energy:* plastic deformation; one or both bones
- *medium energy:* greenstick fracture; one or both bones

Forearm fractures need to be reduced, usually under general anaesthetic, and placed into an above-elbow cast for 3–4 weeks. The reduction is not difficult, but it takes some practice to correct the alignment to neutral and then "crack through" at least one bone's cortex so the angulatory deformity will not quickly recur. Complete healing will take another 4–8 weeks in a short-arm cast, depending on the age of the child.

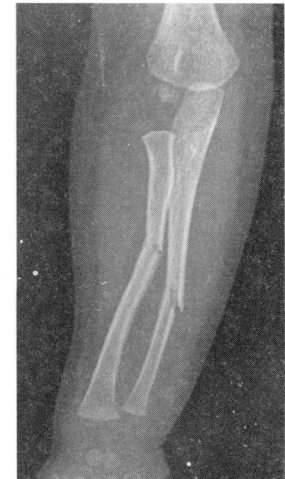

HIGH-ENERGY FOREARM FRACTURES

High-energy forearm fractures comprise two fracture patterns: (a) completely displaced radius and ulna shaft fractures and (b) Monteggia injuries.

Figure 17.3 Greenstick fracture of forearm

Displaced radius and **ulna shaft fractures** are quite tricky to reduce and even harder to maintain the reduction in a cast. These reductions need to be done in the O.R. and often require fixation of one or both bones with a flexible Nancy nail or plate to maintain the reduction. These high-energy forearm shaft fractures are best treated by orthopaedic surgeons from the outset.

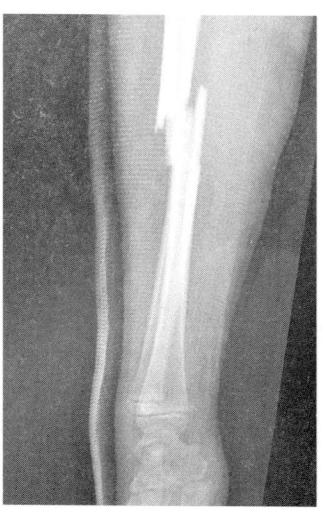
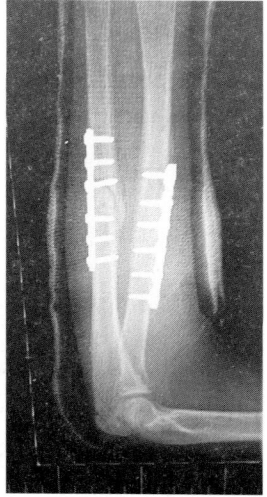

Figure 17.4 Unstable fracture of both radius and ulna treated with plating

The **Monteggia injury** is a variation on the high-energy forearm fracture and presents with a displaced ulnar shaft fracture and dislocated/subluxed radial head. Sometimes the radial head injury is subtle and can be missed. This can be a disaster, as the joint malalignment does not improve with growth and elbow motion can be lost permanently.[2]

It is critical to X-ray the forearm in two planes and to include the joint above and below the injury. The centre of the radial head should line up with the

> The centre of the radial head should line up with the capitellum in every X-ray view of the elbow.

capitellum of the distal lateral humerus in every X-ray view. If this is not the case, then you have a Monteggia injury.

The radial head can sublux or dislocate in various directions, but anteriorly is the most common. The ulnar shaft fracture must be reduced perfectly, and then the radial head will usually reduce. In young children, a closed reduction and cast are sufficient. In older children, usually the ulna needs a plate or flexible pin. Monteggia injuries should always be referred to orthopaedic surgeons.

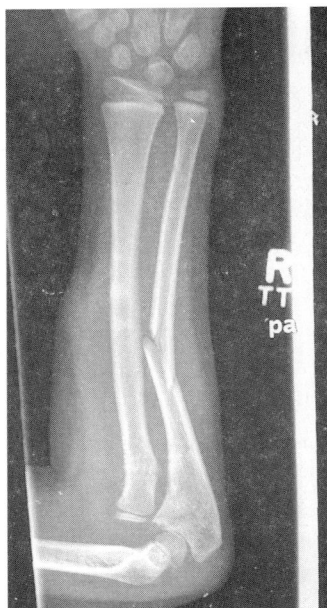 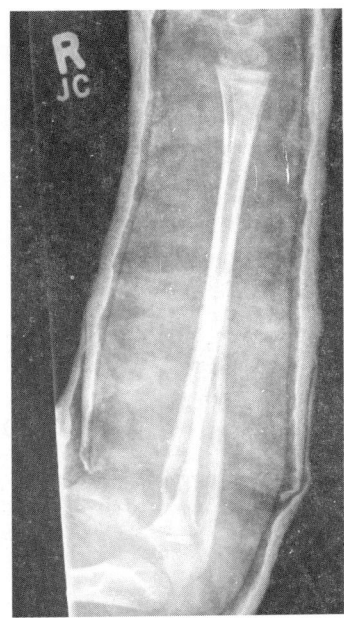

Figure 17.5 Anterior Monteggia injury (Radial head and capitellum do not line up.)

Figure 17.6 Postreduction of same anterior Monteggia injury (Radial head is now aligned with capitellum.)

Ankle and Distal Tibia

Next to wrist and forearm fractures, the ankle is the next most common site of paediatric fracture. The patterns seen are different from the typical malleolar fractures seen in adults — once again, the weak link is in a different location and varies with the age of the child and the amount of energy involved in producing the fracture. The fracture patterns outlined in the following checklist are common.

CHECKLIST OF COMMON ANKLE/DISTAL TIBIA FRACTURES IN CHILDREN

Low energy/younger children
- Salter I injury of fibular growth plate
- varus injury
- lateral swelling/tenderness
- no obvious fracture seen on X-ray
- treatment: 4–6 weeks in weight-bearing cast

Medium energy/younger children/twist
- distal tibial shaft fracture
- does well once realigned
- accept < 5–10 degrees malangulation
- needs above-knee cast for 4 weeks
- then patellar tendon bearing (PTB) or below-knee cast for 6–8 weeks

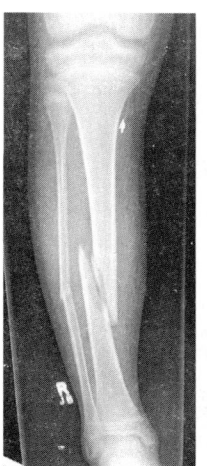 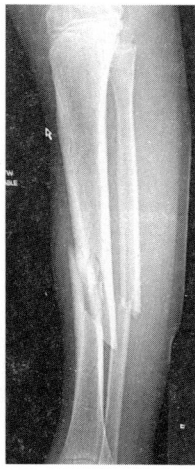 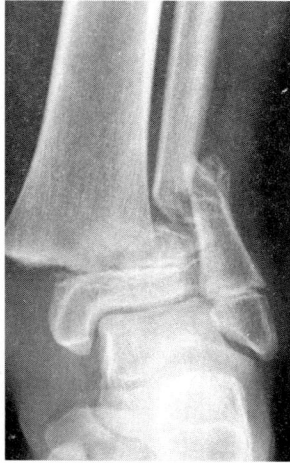

Figure 17.7 Medium-energy tibial shaft fracture in young child

Figure 17.8 Salter II fracture of distal tibia

Medium energy/older children/angular force
- distal tibial growth plate is the weak link in older children
- Salter II distal tibial fracture
- valgus deformities can be impressive
- usually stable once reduced
- easy to reduce in O.R.
- orthopaedic surgeons may supplement with K-wires

Medium energy/older teenagers
- growth plate starting to fuse (medial to lateral and anterior to posterior)
- produces unique weak link where the remaining open physis fails
- predictable fracture pattern considering weak link

Diagnosis and treatment are tricky, so beware of ankle injuries, especially in adolescents. Salter III fractures are intra-articular, so the joint must be perfect. Open reduction is often required.

There are three variations of medium-energy ankle fractures seen in older teenagers: (a) Salter III of the distal lateral tibia (Tillaux fracture), (b) triplane fracture of the distal tibia, and (c) isolated Salter III fracture of the medial malleolus.

SALTER III OF THE DISTAL LATERAL TIBIA (TILLAUX FRACTURE)
This fracture is quite common in the 13- to 16-year age group. The fracture site is very predictable as the weak spot occurs at the open lateral distal tibia growth plate. (The medial side has already started to fuse.) The fracture is intra-articular, so open reduction is the rule.

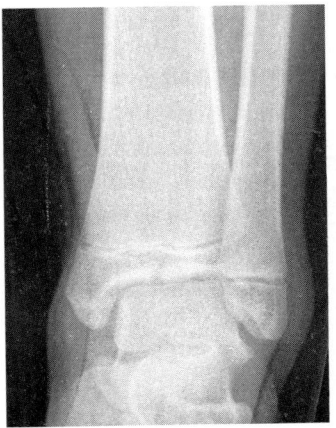

Figure 17.9 Salter III (Tillaux) fracture of distal lateral tibia

TRIPLANE FRACTURE OF THE DISTAL TIBIA
The triplane fracture combines a Salter II distal tibia fracture with a Salter III fracture. These are unusual and tricky to diagnose and treat, even for orthopaedic surgeons. A CT scan can be helpful to determine where the fracture line exits.

ISOLATED SALTER III FRACTURE OF THE MEDIAL MALLEOLUS

An isolated medial malleolus fracture is occasionally seen in older teenagers, just prior to growth plate closure. By definition, it is a Salter III fracture. Usually, these fractures are minimally displaced, but if the joint is not perfect, open reduction is required.

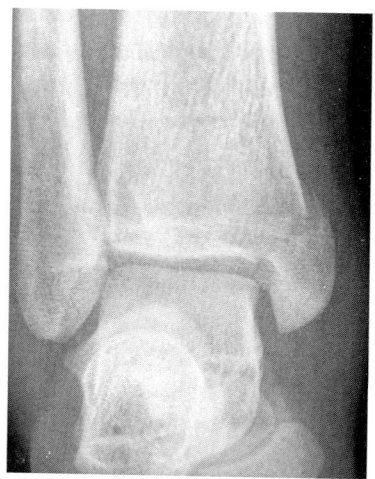

Figure 17.10 Salter III of medial malleolus

REFERENCES

1. Rang M, Pring M., Wenger D. The "slipper" fracture *Fractures in Children*. 3rd ed. Lippincott; 2005. p. 136–7.

2. Ring D, Waters PM. Operative fixation of Monteggia fractures in children. *J Bone Joint Surg Br*. 1996;78(5):734–9. Medline:8836060

18

Most Worrisome Paediatric Fractures: Elbow

Elbow fractures are not the most common of injuries, but they can cause a lot of anxiety among parents and caregivers, both initially, because they swell so much and can affect circulation, and later on, because they can cause growth abnormalities and stiffness.

The elbow becomes vulnerable when children fall, usually backwards, onto a straight arm, or directly onto a flexed elbow. Most of these injuries involve medium- or high-energy falls: (a) trampolines and playground equipment in younger children and (b) bicycles and dirt bikes in older children.

The weak link around the elbow varies with the age of the child. The various secondary growth centres first appear at age 2 and the last at age 12, making diagnosis quite difficult since they can be quite irregular in shape. Whenever in doubt as to what is a fracture line and what is a secondary growth centre, X-ray the opposite elbow as well. Any radiographic variance seen, coupled with point tenderness in that area, is probably a fracture.

> Whenever in doubt as to what is a fracture line and what is a secondary growth centre, X-ray the opposite elbow as well.

Pure dislocations are rare in the elbow joint since the joint capsule is very strong. The exception is an elbow dislocation in a teenager with an associated avulsion of the medial humeral epicondyle.

There are two broad age groups to consider in diagnosis, each with its own characteristic injuries. The following general guidelines are useful.

CHECKLIST OF ELBOW FRACTURES RELATED TO AGE OF CHILD

Young children (3–10 years old)
- growth plates strong; elbow is flexible
- weak link is the metaphyseal bone above or below the elbow (unless high energy, when growth plate can fail, too)
- most common type = supracondylar distal humerus fracture
- less common valgus injury type = radial neck fracture
- least common varus type = Salter IV lateral condyle fracture

Older children (11–16 years old)
- secondary growth centres are weak
- most common type = medial humeral epicondyle fracture
- less common type = olecranon fracture

Supracondylar Distal Humerus Fractures

This is quite a common fracture in younger children involved in high-risk activities, such as falls from furniture at home, climbing equipment at school, or trampolines. Typically, the elbow is quite swollen and the circulation to the fingers may be compromised. Often the fingers are swollen and engorged or purple. In rare cases, they are pale and white, signalling true ischemia.

Temporary nerve injury is also quite common, so a brief neurovascular examination is important. Just as in any fracture, the more displaced the fracture, the more likely there will be an open injury or neurovascular compromise.

The upper limb should be realigned and splinted before moving the child out of the emergency department. This is a gentle realignment, not a reduction of the fracture, and usually means flexing the elbow a little, to improve circulation and lessen the pressure on the soft tissues of the anterior elbow, and then applying an above-elbow posterior half slab. If the hand remains white after this realignment and splinting, which is rare, then you have a true vascular emergency.

The X-rays should confirm the clinical diagnosis. These fractures can be nondisplaced, partially displaced/angulated, or completely displaced with no apposition of the fragments.[1] If undisplaced, the fracture can be splinted and referred to an orthopaedic surgeon for casting within one week; if displaced, definitive reduction must be done under general anaesthetic by an orthopaedic surgeon. The stan-

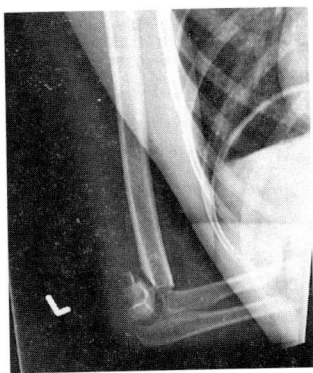 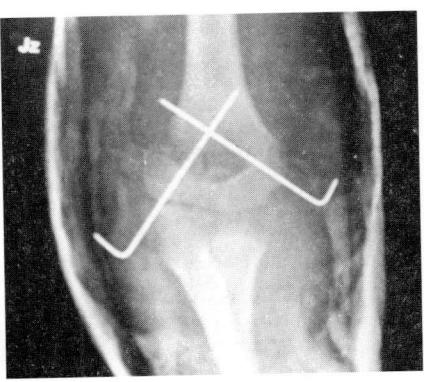

Figure 18.1 Lateral X-ray of a completely displaced supracondylar distal humerus fracture

Figure 18.2 Percutaneous K-wire fixation after closed reduction in the O.R.

dard treatment is a closed reduction and percutaneous pinning since, without pins, these fractures tend to slip once reduced.

Elbow swelling can be a real problem, so the reduction should be done within 6 hours of the injury, not left until the next day. Even without a vascular injury, these little arms are at risk for developing a compartment syndrome if the fracture is displaced, so call the orthopaedic surgeon as soon as you have made your diagnosis and splinted the arm.

Generally, if these fractures are diagnosed, splinted, referred early, and then reduced in the O.R. before the elbow becomes too swollen, then they do very well. The more the initial displacement, the more unstable the fracture will be, and the more difficult the reduction will be to obtain and maintain.

Most community orthopaedic surgeons still find these fractures stressful because the elbow becomes so swollen and because the closed reduction and pinning can be tricky. In addition, in the first week or two after treatment, the fracture reduction can slip around areas of bone comminution or tenuous pin fixation, resulting in an early fracture malposition. Sometimes this occurs in very active children who fall a second time on the elbow while it is still healing. Occasionally, a repeat reduction and pinning are required. Therefore, these fractures are always a challenge.

Partial nerve injury (neuropraxia) is quite common after injury in displaced fractures but usually resolves by 3 months postinjury. Statistically, the anterior interosseous nerve (a branch of the median nerve) is stretched most commonly (more than either the radial nerve or the ulnar nerve).

The postoperative splint is converted to an above-elbow cast at 7–10 days and then casted for a total of 6 weeks. Pins come out after 3–4 weeks.

Even with a great bony reduction and no complications, parents should be warned that the elbow will be stiff for weeks to months after the cast is removed. Physiotherapy is helpful, and no return to rough sports is allowed until the elbow motion is normal.

Other Elbow Fractures in Young Children

RADIAL NECK FRACTURES

This fracture is seen in young children who sustain a valgus strain to the elbow. The fracture through the radial neck can be quite subtle or quite displaced. Angulation up to 30–45 degrees is acceptable, but generally, we try to reduce the angulation in the O.R. with a closed reduction and casting. These elbows need to get moving after 3–4 weeks, especially for forearm rotation.

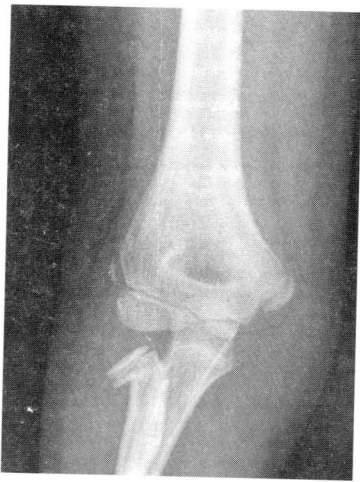

Figure 18.3 Radial neck fracture with valgus angulation

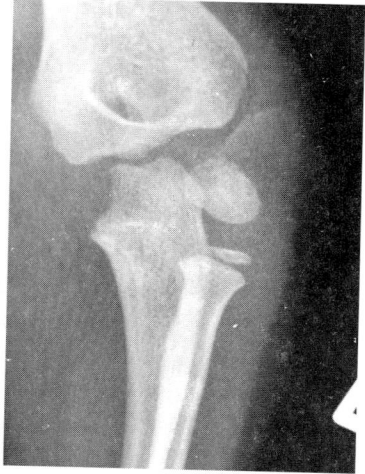

Figure 18.4 X-ray demonstrating a Salter IV lateral condyle fracture (Note how the whole lateral condyle is tilted into varus, right into the joint.)

SALTER IV LATERAL CONDYLE FRACTURES

Fortunately, these fractures are rare, as they involve a lot of varus force on the elbow and go into the elbow joint. Unless the fracture is non-displaced, which is unusual, it must be opened and pinned. The growth plate and joint are involved, so these can lead to chronic elbow stiffness and growth arrest problems.

PULLED ELBOW

This is a relatively common condition seen in young children in the 1- to 3-year age group who present to the office or emergency department with pain and inability to flex their elbow after a minor traumatic event.

Typically, a pulled elbow occurs when a small child is walking with an uplifted arm holding a parent's hand. When the child lags behind or misbehaves, the parent pulls forcefully on the child's uplifted and extended arm, the elbow is injured, and the child starts to cry. There is no swelling or deformity at the elbow, but the child holds the affected arm straight and will not flex it.

The presentation is quite classic in this age group. Anatomically, the flexible annular ligament of the lateral elbow has subluxed over the radial head in extension and pronation. X-rays will be normal.

Treatment consists of gently and passively flexing and supinating the affected elbow past 90 degrees of flexion. Often the elbow will click and the child will immediately stop crying. Sometimes this can occur in the X-ray department when the technician flexes the elbow for the lateral X-ray view. No further treatment is needed once the elbow becomes asymptomatic.

Occasionally, orthopaedic surgeons are consulted because the pulled elbow does not respond to flexing past 90 degrees, and the child remains unhappy.

These little elbows should be placed in an above-elbow half splint in 90 degrees of flexion and as much supination as possible, to be worn 24 hours per day for 3–5 days. This treatment settles down the muscle spasm and allows the annular ligament to slowly slide back into its normal position around the radial neck.

Once the half splint is removed, the child's elbow is usually painless with full active motion. No further treatment is required, apart from preventative counselling for the parents.

Elbow Fractures in Older Children

MEDIAL EPICONDYLE DISTAL HUMERUS FRACTURES

This is a common injury with a valgus strain to the elbow in older teenagers. The fracture may be minimally displaced, displaced more than 1 cm, or stuck in the elbow joint after it dislocated and was reduced. The ulnar nerve is right in the injury zone and is often contused but rarely damaged permanently. Surgery is indicated if the medial epicondyle is displaced more than 5–10 mm, the nerve is out, or the fragment is entrapped in the joint. Open reduction and pinning is required.

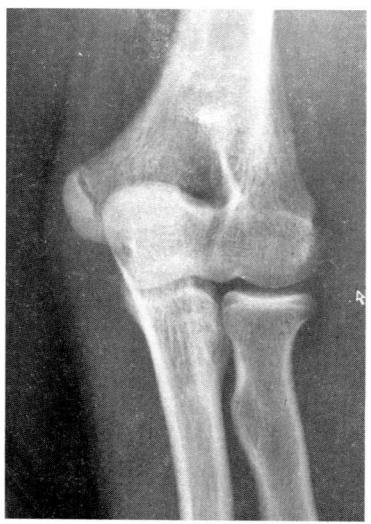

Figure 18.5 Medial epicondyle fracture (minimally displaced)

OLECRANON FRACTURES

These fractures are not common in children. Older teenagers sometimes present with this fracture after a fall onto a flexed elbow. The secondary growth centre of the olecranon can be a weak link. If the fracture is displaced more than 5 mm, and if the child cannot actively extend the elbow against gravity, then open reduction and fixation is indicated.

REFERENCE
1. Hed J, Bould M, Livingstone J, et al. Reproducibility of the Gartland classification for supracondylar humerus fractures in children. *J Orthop Surg.* 2007;15(1):12–4.

19

Remaining Paediatric Fractures by Region

Clavicle

Most clavicle injuries do extremely well with nonoperative treatment. Despite the appearance of the initial X-rays, these will heal. Simple sling and swath immobilization for comfort is all that is needed for 3–4 weeks. It is really quite amazing to see how clavicle fractures fill in with abundant fracture callus within a few weeks, especially in younger children.

Except for an open injury, there is almost no need to treat a clavicle fracture in a child operatively. In older teenagers, the temptation to operate is greater, but mid-shaft fractures still usually heal without surgery, possibly taking up to 3 months, as in an adult.

A variant of AC joint separation is seen in teenagers, where the distal clavicle growth plate separates and remains with the acromion, and the clavicle displaces medially. The deformity looks quite bad, but these will also heal without surgery with abundant callus.

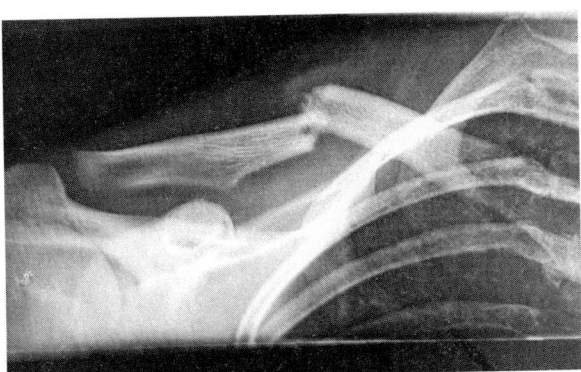

Figure 19.1 Clavicle fracture in an adolescent (This will heal and round off nicely.)

Shoulder/Humerus

Shoulder fractures in children do very well. The shoulder has a large arc of normal motion, so angulation of up to 45 degrees is well tolerated. In addition, 80% of the growth of the humerus occurs at the proximal end, so these fractures remodel quickly. Three fracture patterns are commonly seen in children: (a) metaphyseal (impacted) fractures, (b) Salter II proximal humerus fractures, and (c) humeral shaft fractures.

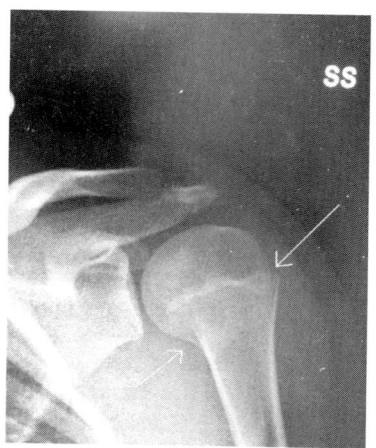

Figure 19.2 Salter II of proximal humerus impacted

METAPHYSEAL (IMPACTED) FRACTURES

These are common in younger children with sturdy growth plates. Some varus angulation may be present, usually less than 30 degrees. Treatment is conservative, with sling and swath for 3 weeks, followed by physiotherapy. The fracture is generally healed in 6 weeks. Rough sports should be avoided for 3 months.

A variation seen in older children is the metaphyseal fracture through a benign unicameral bone cyst. This is a relatively common site of fracture. Though the X-rays look dramatic, the fracture will heal with the same treatment as previously mentioned. The bone cyst usually fills in with bone after the fracture, but it may take 6–12 months to do so. Orthopaedic consultation is usually prudent in these cases.

SALTER II PROXIMAL HUMERUS FRACTURES

In older children, these fractures are seen in high-energy injuries, such as falling off a horse, and are more common in girls, probably due to less muscle bulk. Angulation can be quite impressive and, because these girls are often slim, the deformity is obvious (typically into varus and with the fracture apex anterior). The growth plate of the proximal humerus is irregularly shaped, like a circus tent, so diagnosis of the fracture line path can be confusing.

Although these fractures will heal and remodel well, generally, if more than 20–30 degrees of angulation is present, they should be referred for closed reduction in the O.R. Because the fractures can be unstable after reduction, orthopaedic surgeons now routinely percutaneously pin these fractures for 3 weeks.

HUMERAL SHAFT FRACTURES

These are uncommon in children, since the shaft is strong and elastic, but a direct blow may cause such a fracture. Treatment is conservative: use a sugar-tong splint for 4–6 weeks and extreme caution in sports for 3 months.

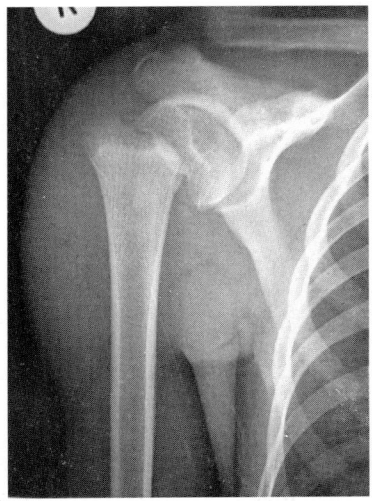

Figure 19.3 Salter II fracture of proximal humerus

Femur

Hip fractures are rare in children, but fractures of the femoral shaft are not uncommon. The femoral shaft is a large, strong bone, so a lot of force is required to fracture it. In young children, especially those younger than 3 years of age, a fractured femur can be a red flag for child abuse, so a de-

> In young children, a fractured femur can be a red flag for child abuse.

tailed accident history should be obtained. If there are any inconsistencies in the story, a full skeletal survey should be ordered, and the social work team should be involved.

Femur fractures will heal with traction and casting. Historically, children were kept in the hospital for weeks in traction until the fracture was "sticky enough" not to slip when placed into a cast. This is still done in the developing world. Unfortunately, a fractured femur can take up to 6–8 weeks before it will not slip in a cast. The modern trend in orthopaedics is to discharge the child home as soon as possible. This can be facilitated in the O.R. by early hip spica casting and the use of removable flexible fixation nails, which do not violate the growth plates.

Femoral shaft fractures should be referred to orthopaedic surgeons and, when possible, to paediatric subspecialists, since flexible nailing is not done by all community orthopaedic surgeons. The goal is to have the fracture healed within the following parameters:

- less than 5 degrees varus/valgus
- less than 10 degrees anterior/posterior bow
- less than 1 cm shortening (Some overgrowth will occur with healing.)
- no malrotation

Femur fracture healing time is directly correlated with the child's age. This can vary between 6–8 weeks in toddlers to up to 4–6 months in teenagers. The overall average would be 3–4 months. Treatment is, therefore, dictated primarily by the age of the child, as outlined in the following checklist.

CHECKLIST OF FEMUR FRACTURE TREATMENT BY AGE
0–36 months old
- immediate hip spica application in O.R.; or skin traction x days then hip spica in O.R.

3–8 years of age
- period of days to 2 weeks in traction (skin or skeletal)

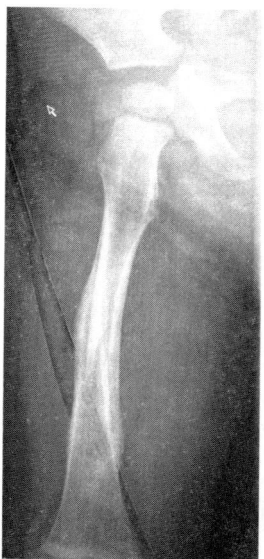 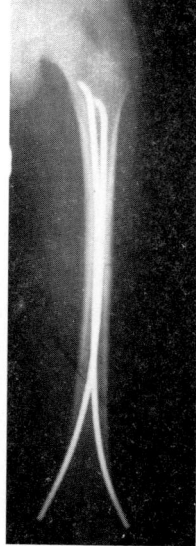 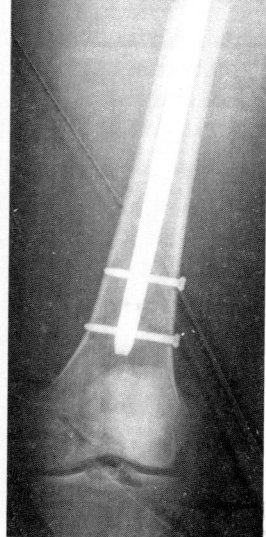

Figure 19.4 Healing mid-shaft femur fracture in a toddler

Figure 19.5 Flexible nailing of femoral shaft fracture

Figure 19.6 Standard intramedullary femoral shaft nailing in older teenager

- hip spica cast or flexible nails with hip spica
- trend toward getting children out of traction, and out of hospital, earlier, so age of flexible nailing is steadily declining

8–14 years of age
- immediate flexible nailing and spica casting
- older than 14 years (or child with closed growth plates) requires immediate standard intramedullary nailing (as in adults)

DISTAL FEMUR FRACTURES (SALTER II)

This is an uncommon, but important, fracture because 70% of the growth of the femur occurs at its distal end. Fractures here can produce growth arrest. This area becomes the weak link only in older teenagers, usually boys, when they are involved in high-risk sports and are struck in the knee area with a valgus or varus force, an injury that would cause a knee ligament injury in a skeletally mature patient.

Treatment involves closed reduction in the O.R. The fracture can be unstable, so the reduction is usually supple-

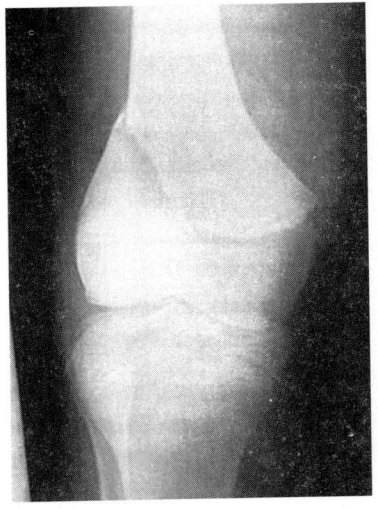

Figure 19.7 Salter II distal femur fracture

mented with percutaneous pins or screws and a long leg cast. Healing time is 8–12 weeks. Due to the shear forces across the physis, premature growth arrest can occur, and these fractures should be watched for several years.

Knee Injuries

Unlike adults, knee injuries are not common in children. In particular, knee ligament injuries are rare, as the ligaments are not the weak link in this age group. A few classic injuries are seen, however: (a) metaphyseal proximal tibia fractures, (b) tibial spine and tubercle injuries, and (c) patellar dislocations.

METAPHYSEAL PROXIMAL TIBIA FRACTURES

These fractures are seen in young children, usually younger than 10 years of age, and involve a valgus injury to the tibial plateau. They can drift into valgus with healing, so they should be reduced into neutral alignment if any valgus is present initially. Treatment involves a non-weight-bearing, above-knee cast for 3 weeks followed by a weight-bearing cast for another 3 weeks.

TIBIAL SPINE AND TUBERCLE INJURIES

These injuries occur in older children, around 8–12 years, when the ACL avulses a bony fragment from the tibia. (The bone is the weak link.) If displaced, these must be repaired.

Treatment involves pulling down the tibial spine and anchoring it back to the tibia. Above-knee splinting/casting is needed for 6–8 weeks. These fractures do well if repaired; the knee becomes lax if the displaced fragment is left unrepaired.

PATELLAR DISLOCATIONS

Patellar dislocations are common injuries, particularly in adolescent girls with flexible joints. The patellar always dislocates laterally and often is reduced "on the field" as soon as the girl fully extends her knee. The swelling can be quite impressive and the anxiety level high.

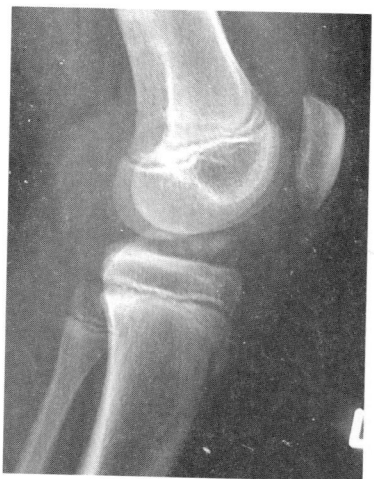

Figure 19.8 Tibial spine fracture (ACL has been avulsed.)

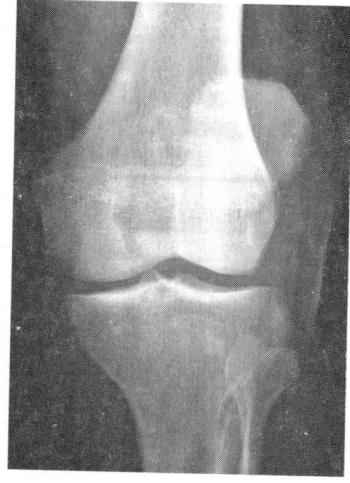

Figure 19.9 Lateral patellar dislocation

X-rays should rule out a large osteochondral fragment, which occasionally flakes off the lateral femoral condyle or the medial patellar facet. If present, an urgent referral for an arthroscopy should be obtained to remove the loose body.

Generally, treatment is conservative: splint and crutches for 3–4 weeks followed by physiotherapy. If the girl has a valgus knee and lax joints, the dislocation may be recurrent, and orthopaedic elective referral may help.

Foot

Foot fractures are quite uncommon in children. Usually they are the result of a crush injury and involve the metatarsals and toes. Displacement is usually minimal due to the excellent periosteal coverings of the bones. Treatment requires a non-weight-bearing splint for 3 weeks followed by a weight-bearing cast for another 3 weeks.

Spine

Children are flexible and relatively short, so the spine is only at risk in very high-energy trauma situations. Children in these circumstances will likely be transferred to dedicated trauma centres directly from the scene of the accident. Any fracture is possible with enough force, but fortunately, these are rare injuries.

Pelvis

These are also rare injuries, only seen in a multiple trauma situation. The pelvic ligaments are more flexible in children than in adults, so fractures are rare. However, there is one variation of pelvic injuries not associated with high-energy trauma that is seen occasionally in community practice: the avulsion of iliac spines.

AVULSION OF ILIAC SPINES FROM PELVIS (OR HIP)

This variation of pelvis injury is sometimes seen in very active teenagers, boys more than girls, involved in such sports as hockey, track and field, or dance. The injury occurs when an extreme stretch pulls the muscle attachment off the apophysis in the ASIS, AIIS, or greater or lesser trochanter. Treatment is conservative, with crutches and physiotherapy, and abstaining from sports for 4–8 weeks. Please see Chapter 27 for more details about this overuse type of injury.

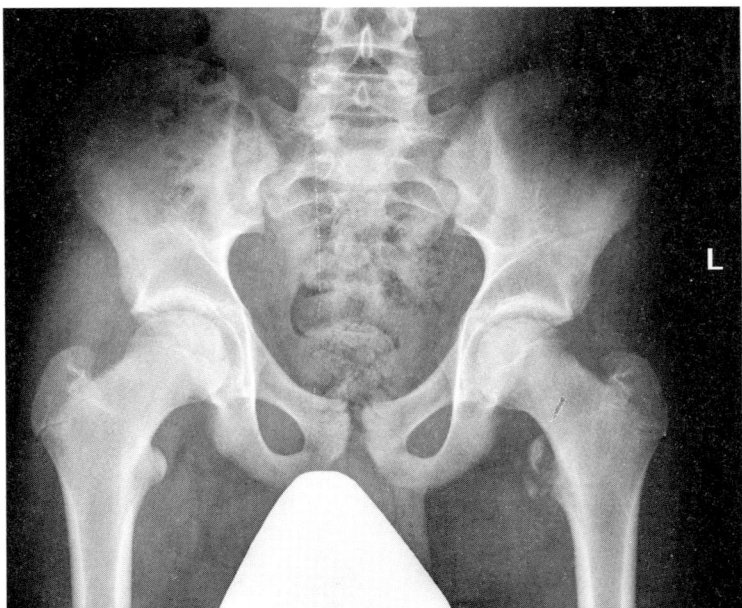

Figure 19.10 Avulsion fracture of the left lesser trochanter of hip

Conclusion: Paediatric Fractures

Children's fractures generally do well, with a few caveats: (a) treat su-pracondylar distal humerus fractures with great respect; (b) remem-ber that children's fractures heal quickly and are "stuck where the position lies" by 2 weeks, and that every fracture will not "remodel"; and finally, (c) refer the high-energy, unstable fracture pattern injuries to orthopaedic surgeons early rather than struggling to treat every in-jury seen in children in the primary-care setting.

PART FOUR

ELECTIVE ORTHOPAEDICS IN ADULTS

20

Overview

Many orthopaedic disorders are seen electively in the office. Ortho-paedic specialists receive the most complaints from family doctors about the inordinately long waits for consultation for patients com-plaining of disability. Stiffness, instability, and pain are not life or limb threatening, but they do cause a great deal of disability. Unfortunately, in Canada, patients often wait months, or even years, to see an ortho-paedic specialist for conditions in this general group; then they may be placed on a waiting list for surgery and again have to wait several months. Obviously, this is not ideal and is one of the biggest criticisms of the Canadian health care system.

Disorders will be presented according to their relative incidence of presentation to a community-based orthopaedic surgeon, on an ana-tomical basis:

- knee disorders
- shoulder disorders
- hip and low back disorders
- foot and ankle disorders
- hand, wrist, and elbow disorders

Once seen by an orthopaedic specialist, probably less than one-third to one-half of patients will clearly benefit from surgery at the

time of the initial visit. Many patients require more time for conservative modalities or have levels
of disability that do not yet
warrant surgical intervention. Others may benefit
from surgery but are medically unfit for the procedure.

> In general, younger patients tend to present with painful and unstable joints and older patients with painful and stiff joints. This applies to most anatomic areas.

Every case is different and must balance the risks and benefits of surgery with conservative modalities.

If operative treatment is indicated, *several operative interventions* are possible for every joint. In general, they follow in increasing order of aggressiveness:

- *arthroscopy:* (debridement and repairs)
  - most common procedures performed in orthopaedics
  - almost any major joint can be arthroscoped

- *open debridement:* (decompressions and repairs)
  - nerve releases, open joint repairs
  - large joint debridements for infection (implants)

- *arthroplasty:* highly successful in hip and knee; very common
  - replacement (hip, knee, shoulder, elbow, possibly ankle)
  - interposition (soft tissue in the wrist and elbow)

- *fusion:* as default procedure for arthritic joints (foot and ankle, wrist)
- *amputation:*
  - last-resort procedure for failed less invasive procedures

21

Knee

Up to 50% of visits to a general orthopaedic clinic are for problems related to the knee joint.[1] All age groups may be involved, but the disorders can be broadly separated into two groups: (a) younger patients with problems of global or patellar instability, or with locking symptoms and (b) older patients with swelling and locking or pain and stiffness.

YOUNGER PATIENTS	OLDER PATIENTS (OLDER THAN 40)
• instability: global or patellar • locking symptoms	• swelling and locking • pain and stiffness

Younger Patients

WITH INSTABILITY

History-taking is very important in this subgroup of knee patients. They are generally young, athletic people who have intermittent problems with their knee in certain activities or sports. Usually there has been a sports-related knee injury in the past. Two patterns of instability are common: patellar and global.

PATELLAR

- older teenagers and young adults; mostly girls; kneecap pops laterally with unstable event
- *exam:* look for valgus; ligament laxity generally; positive apprehension with lateral patellar force
- *treatment:* soft brace; physiotherapy; arthroscopic lavage/release
- patellar realignment (Maquet, etc.) if kneecap has popped more than three times

GLOBAL INSTABILITY (ACL; MCL; COMBINED; VARIANTS)

These patients have a history of a significant knee injury in the past.

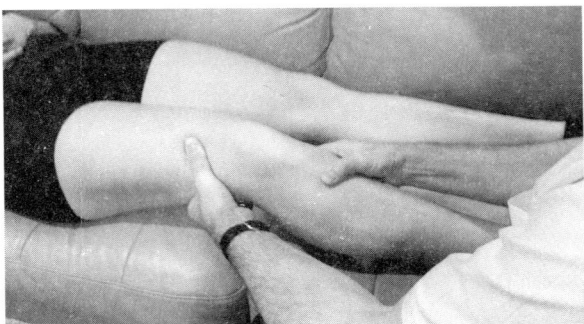

Figure 21.1 Lachman test: must be on same side as affected knee when examining

Usually the knee was very swollen at the time and then was never quite the same. These patients have lost confidence in their knee; it gives way when turning corners, when running, or when stopping suddenly. The knee may also lock briefly. Running in a straight line is often okay. Ask about investigations and treatments to date.

Physical exam (compare to normal, contralateral knee):

- MCL
- LCL stress
- Lachman test
- joint line tenderness

An MRI is very useful in this subgroup of patients before proceeding with any surgery (R/O meniscal injury; posterior capsular pathology).

Treatment should start with physiotherapy, sport modification, and bracing. For many active patients, ACL reconstruction is usually the best option, but the timing of surgery is controversial.[2] Most centres have surgeons with an interest in sports medicine and patients should ultimately be referred to these ACL surgeons.

WITH LOCKING

This group of patients presents primarily with locking sensations. They often present acutely to the emergency department with a locked knee, but on questioning, usually have a long history of locking episodes. These people have difficulty kneeling or getting up after crouching. Often they cannot fully extend their knee.

Differential diagnosis: medial meniscal (bucket-handle tear); lateral meniscal tear (often in ACL-deficient knees); or a loose body from OCD.

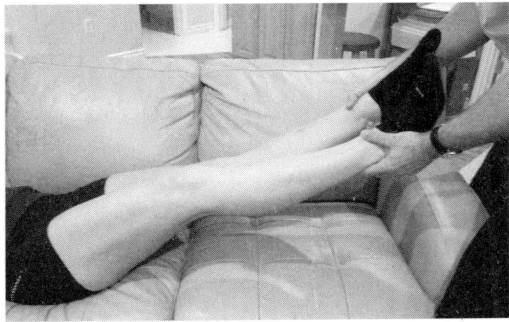

Figure 21.2 Note the lack of full right knee extension (classic finding in a bucket-handle meniscal tear).

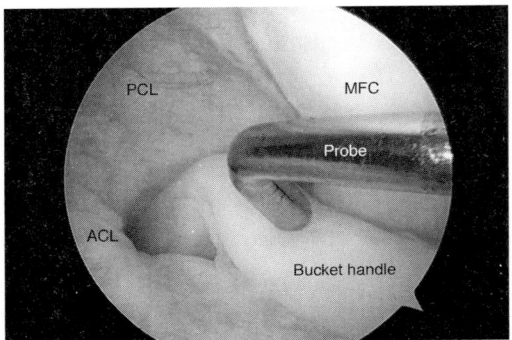

Figure 21.3 Bucket-handle tear of medial meniscus

Treatment would be expedited arthroscopy, usually to excise the offending fragment, sometimes to repair the meniscus.

Older Patients

WITH SWELLING AND LOCKING

A swelling and locking knee in the older patient is a very common presentation to the office. These generally healthy people have few symptoms with their knee until they "overdo it"; for example, they increase their jogging mileage, play in a weekend baseball tournament, or start home renovations. As they age, the trend for more of these flare-ups increases.

The physical exam shows joint line tenderness and often crepitus over the patellofemoral or medial compartment. X-rays are usually normal or show mild joint space narrowing.

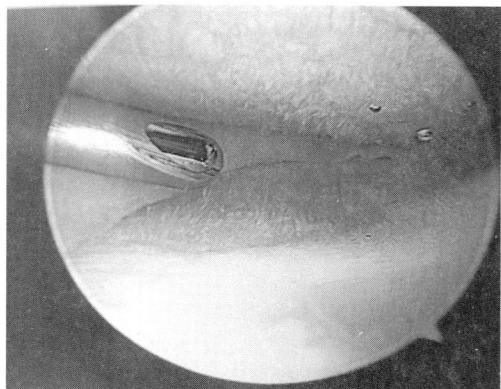

Figure 21.4 Arthroscopic appearance of degenerative medial knee joint space

Treatment involves the usual NSAID, weight loss, or sport modification, if applicable. One or two Depo-Medrol injections are helpful for flare-ups. Arthroscopic lavage/debridement is widely done for this condition. At surgery, one finds degenerative meniscal tears/debris (usually medial) and deep chondromalacia or early osteoarthritis of the medial, patellofemoral, and lateral compartments.

Most general community orthopaedic surgeons will do several of these cases per week week with gratifying results for patients for 2–5 years, although some recent literature contradicts this.[3] For most of us, it remains one of the best operations we can offer patients.

WITH PAIN AND STIFFNESS

This group of patients has constant and progressive symptoms. The pain is deep, aching, and made worse by walking, kneeling, or going up and down stairs. Most of these patients are older than 60 years of age, but middle-aged patients can present if they have had previous knee injuries or surgery.

Ask about the following:

- analgesic use
- need for a cane
- pain at night
- distance that can be walked before patient must stop

Most surgeons will not consider replacement arthroplasty in patients who do not need a cane.

PHYSICAL EXAM

- check knee alignment (varus > valgus)
- measure motion (best predictor of postoperative ROM)

Plain X-rays are the correct diagnostic tool in these cases. An MRI is *not* helpful in this patient group. On the X-rays, look for joint space narrowing and its pattern, for osteophyte formation, and for any joint malalignment. Patterns seen include the following:

- varus knee (medial alone); may be candidate for unicompartment replacement
- varus knee (medial > patellofemoral > lateral joint); most common pattern seen; total knee replacement only option
- valgus knee (often rheumatoid) = total knee replacement best option
- isolated patellofemoral; patellar replacement alone = Avon type versus TKR

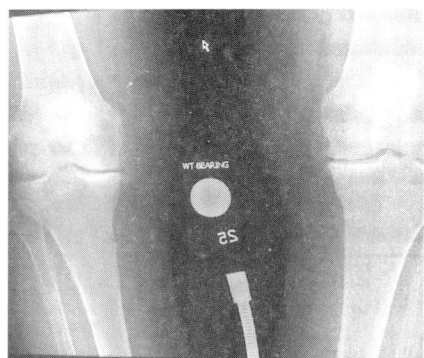

Figure 21.5 Isolated medial O/A

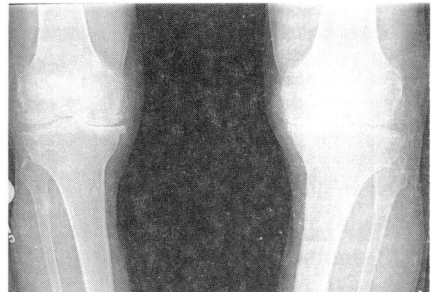

Figure 21.6 More advanced global knee arthritis

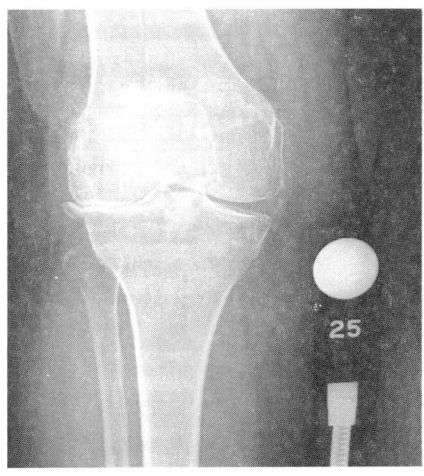

Figure 21.7 Valgus knee (often rheumatoid arthritis)

CHECKLIST OF SURGICAL OPTIONS FOR KNEE DISORDERS

- arthroscopic lavage (if too young or not symptomatic enough for TKR)
- osteotomy (if young and isolated varus or valgus = unusual)
- replacement arthroplasty (unicompartment or full replacement)

Total knee replacement results

- patient selection important
- older than 55 years of age (retired or semiretired with light-duty work)
- ADL compromised
- failure of previous modalities
- circulation okay
- obese? (not ideal, but increasingly common)
- reasonable lifestyle/compliant
- no contraindications (infection; neuromotor imbalance)
- very good results in most patients, but not universally as good as with total hip replacements due to persistent pain or knee stiffness

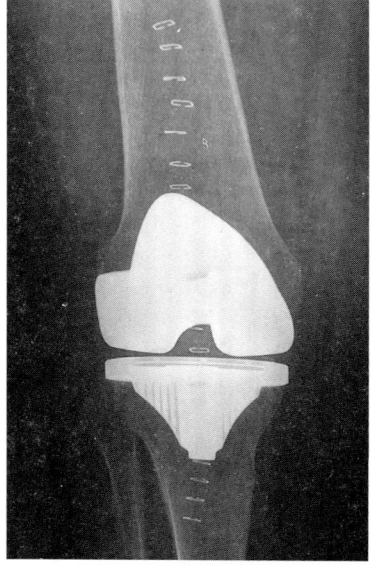

Figure 21.8 Tricompartmental total knee replacement (tibia, femur, patella)

REFERENCES

1. Woolf AD, Pfleger B. Burden of major musculoskeletal conditions. *Bull World Health Organ.* 2003;81(9):646–56. Medline:14710506

2. Wasilewski SA, Covall DJ, Cohen S. Effect of surgical timing on recovery and associated injuries after anterior cruciate ligament reconstruction. *Am J Sports Med.* 1993;21(3):338–42. http://dx.doi.org/10.1177/036354659302100302. Medline:8346744

3. Kirkley A, Birmingham TB, Litchfield RB, et al. A randomized trial of arthroscopic surgery for osteoarthritis of the knee. *N Engl J Med.* 2008;359(11):1097–107. http://dx.doi.org/10.1056/NEJMoa0708333. Medline:18784099

22

Shoulder

After knee disorders, shoulder problems are probably the most frequently encountered in the office setting. All age groups can be involved and like the knee, the disorders can be grouped broadly by age: (a) younger patients with pain and instability symptoms and (b) older patients with pain and weakness/stiffness.

Younger Patients

Patients less than 35 years of age generally have intermittent and activity-related symptoms. Overhead activities are the most problematic: throwing a ball, front crawl swimming, or stretching overhead or away from the body to make a play. The pain is sudden, catching, and may make the arm "feel dead" for a while. There may be a distant history of an injury, especially with frank dislocations or, more commonly, a progressive trend to more symptoms as the dedication to the sport increased.

The differential diagnosis in this age group includes the following:

- glenohumeral joint instability (traumatic versus habitual)
- A/C joint injury with impingement
- labral tears
- superior labral anterio posterior (SLAP) tears (biceps insertion lesions)

Rotator cuff tears, per se, are rare in this age group. The cuff can be thickened but rarely tears completely (unlike in the older age group).

The physical exam, in concert with the history, is usually diagnostic. Look for impingement, joint laxity (local and generalized), and apprehension tests (see Chapter 2).

Plain X-rays often appear normal in this age group, but an MRI can be very useful in detecting even small tears around the shoulder.

The basic questions are (a) where is the lesion? and (b) is it traumatic or habitual?

Physiotherapy can be very helpful, especially for those patients with generalized ligamentous laxity and unstable shoulders.

Shoulder arthroscopy by a surgeon who specializes in sports medicine can be diagnostic and curative if the lesion is amenable to arthroscopic repair. Open repairs, particularly for recurrent anterior traumatic shoulder dislocators, still have a good success rate.[1]

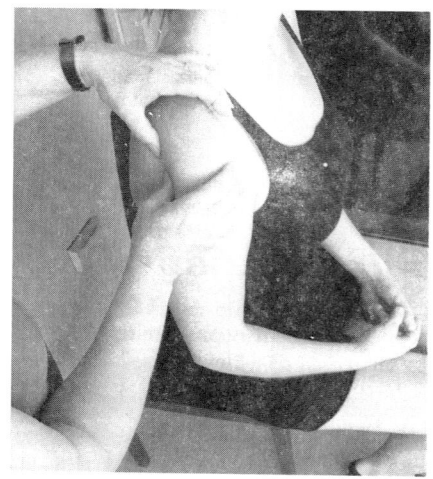

Figure 22.1 Shoulder passive subluxation testing

Older Patients (Older Than Age 45)

Patients older than 45 years of age often arrive at the office electively with shoulder complaints. They generally present with an "acute on chronic" history of shoulder pain with overhead activities. Symptoms are brought on by repetitive use overhead, a minor fall on the extended shoulder, or an unexpected strain to the extended shoulder. The loss to elevation strength can be gradual or sudden and profound (if the tear is complete and large).

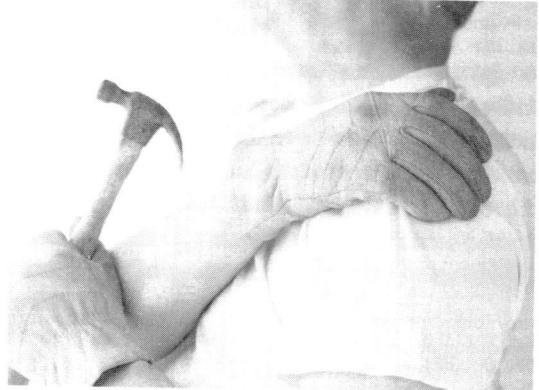

Figure 22.2 Classic history for overuse shoulder disorders

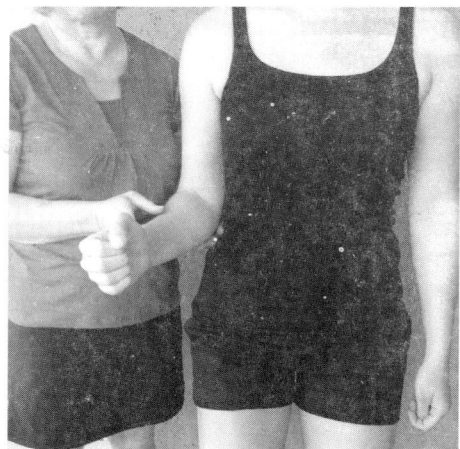

Figure 22.3 Rotator cuff: infraspinatus test

Ask about the following:

- handedness
- ADL, especially overhead activities
- night pain: very common and classic for shoulder disorders
- analgesic use

The physical exam should document ROM, crepitus, and rotator cuff strength (see Chapter 2).

All these patients have "impingement syndrome," which broadly includes many diagnostic conditions including tendonitis, cuff tears, arthritis, and frozen shoulder. Answer the following questions before selecting treatment:

- Is there a rotator cuff tear present?
- Is it partial or complete?
- Is there AC joint arthritis?
- Is there glenohumeral joint arthritis? (poor shoulder rotation and older patients typically)

Plain X-rays will show the AC joint and glenohumeral joint nicely. (Most of these patients have normal glenohumeral joints.) A shoulder ultrasound is a quick, inexpensive test to determine if a cuff tear is present and whether it is partial or complete. An MRI is rarely needed in this age group to determine treatment.

CHECKLIST OF TREATMENT OPTIONS FOR IMPINGEMENT SYNDROME

Impingement alone with no cuff tears

- NSAID
- physiotherapy
- pulleys at home
- Depo-Medrol into subacromial space
- failure to improve = arthroscopic debridement

Impingement with partial cuff tear (and fair to good cuff strength)

- as above + book arthroscopic debridement sooner

Impingement with complete cuff tear (and poor cuff strength)

- expedited cuff repair (arthroscopic or open = surgeon dependent)

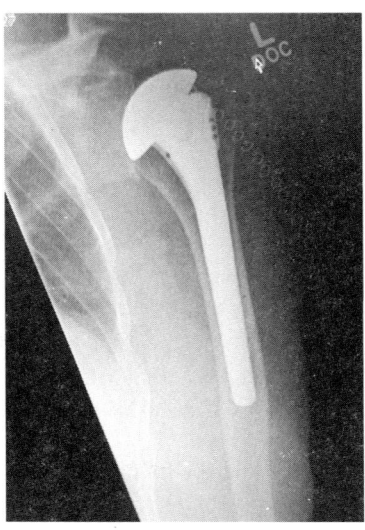

Figure 22.4 Shoulder hemiarthroplasty for cuff arthropathy

Impingement with glenohumeral joint arthritis

- conservative modalities until failure; then arthroplasty (hemi- or total shoulder arthroplasty)
- arthroscopic modalities not very effective in this group

REFERENCE

1. Cole BJ, Warner JJP. Arthroscopic versus open Bankart repair for traumatic anterior shoulder instability. *Clin Sports Med.* 2000;19(1):19–48. http://dx.doi.org/10.1016/S0278-5919(05)70294-5. Medline:10652663

23

Hip and Low Back

Particularly in the older age group, it is often difficult to separate pain originating from the hip from pain originating in the low back, so the two will be discussed together. Many elderly patients with bad hip arthritis also have relatively severe degenerative lumbar spinal problems that can contribute to their symptoms.

Older Patients (Older Than Age 60)

Those older than 60 years of age form the largest group of patients who present with groin and buttock pain. Generally, the pain has been present for years and is slowly worsening. Pain is worse at night and worsens with walking and with the first few steps after sitting. Stiffness is a prominent feature. If patients have associated leg numbness and need to sit down for pain relief (not just stop walking), look for **lumbar spinal stenosis** as well.

HISTORY
Ask about the following:

- analgesic use
- need for a cane
- difficulty putting on shoes and socks

PHYSICAL EXAM

- watch gait (Trendelenburg)
- check hip ROM (Patients lose internal rotation and flexion first.)
- leg shortening?
- check L-spine ROM
- neurologic exam
- knee ROM

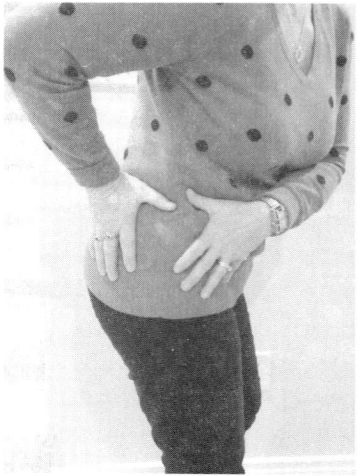

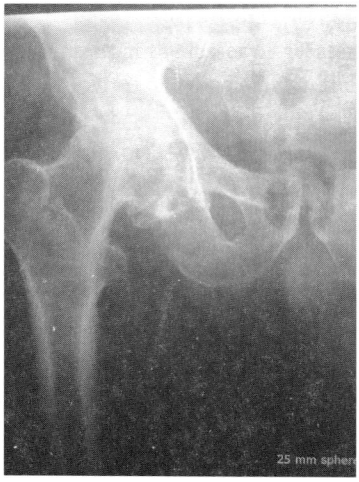

Figure 23.1 Common location of hip pain

Figure 23.2 O/A of right hip with severe loss of joint space

- plain X-ray: AP pelvis (shows both hips; SI joints; lower L-spine) affected hip
- CT lumbar spine (if suspecting associated spinal stenosis)

For most patients with this presentation, the only reasonable surgical treatment is total hip arthroplasty, except in the spinal stenosis group. The question becomes "is the patient ready for THR?" In Canada, most patients wait so long for their initial consultation with an orthopaedic surgeon that they are only too willing to proceed with surgical booking at that time.

CHECKLIST OF GENERAL INDICATIONS FOR HIP REPLACEMENT

Indications

- advanced stage arthritis on X-ray
- older/more sedentary/compliant
- regular analgesic required
- failure of conservative modalities
- decrease in ADL; usually use of a cane required

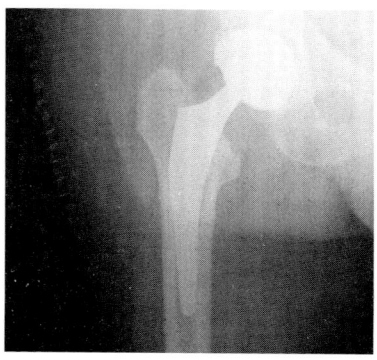

Figure 23.3 Uncemented right THR

Relative contraindications
- young patients with physically demanding jobs
- morbid obesity
- significant medical co-morbidities
- sometimes done if there are no other reasonable surgical options

Absolute contraindications
- infection
- neuromuscular imbalance

Many patients with borderline indications or high risk factors are simply told to wait, and we follow them every 6 months in the clinic.

There is great discussion about what type of implant is best for each patient. Fads come and go every 5–10 years, especially for the young patient with hip arthritis. For older patients, a metal on plastic hybrid or uncemented THR is the standard of care and should last 15–20 years.

Outcomes for THR, in the right patient population, are excellent. Pain relief is almost immediate and ADL improvement is dramatic.[1]

Governments are now setting standards for wait times for THR procedures in Canada. The goal is to have the surgery performed within 3–6 months after consultation with the orthopaedic surgeon. The problem is still the delay in getting the first consultation.

Younger Patients

Hip Pain

The diagnosis in the younger age group is usually not difficult to determine and usually only one hip joint is involved. The problem is what to do for patients who are at high risk for failure with traditional THR. The usual predisposing factors are as follows:

- childhood hip disorders (DDH; Perthes; SCFE; infection)
- hip/pelvic trauma as a young adult
- AVN: post-traumatic; steroid use; postradiation; alcoholism; idiopathic
- inflammatory arthritis: rheumatoid; ankylosing spondylitis

Most orthopaedic surgeons follow these patients along nonoperatively for as long as possible before performing the inevitable THR. Newer technologies for hip replacement in this younger, higher-risk group are becoming available. These tend to preserve more bone than traditional THR or use different bearing surfaces. Therefore, these younger patients should be referred to an orthopaedic surgeon in the community who has some experience with these new technologies.

Back Pain

The younger patient who presents with back and leg pain is easier to sort out than the elderly patient with back and buttock/leg pain. These younger patients rarely have pathology in their hips or circulatory problems in their lower limbs, unlike the elderly population.

It is helpful to separate back pain into two categories[2]: (a) back pain dominant (local spinal segment pain) and (b) leg pain dominant (nerve root pain).

BACK PAIN DOMINANT

This is the most common presentation to the office. There is a large potential differential diagnosis, but typically, most cases are called **mechanical back pain (or lumbago)**.

The pain arises from the lumbar disc/facet complex and is degenerative in nature. The episodes develop suddenly, often after relative overuse of the lower spine. The pain is lower lumbar and central, rarely radiating past the buttocks, and is generally better with the extension of the spine. Episodes last a few days to one or two weeks and there are no neurologic findings.

Plain X-rays show as normal or with an early DJD spinal segment (narrowed disc space; facet enlargement at lower lumbar spine). A CT scan confirms degenerative spinal segment changes, but neural elements are usually normal.

Treatment should be conservative. Lumbar exercises are very important after a flare-up in order to prevent recurrence.[3] If the patient shows a trend to recurrent flare-ups despite being compliant with the back exercise program, he or she may benefit from a local lumbar fusion (fewer than 5% of patients).

In the small group of patients with dominant back pain who do not fit this usual pattern of symptoms and response to treatment, consider the full differential diagnosis of back pain.

DIFFERENTIAL DIAGNOSIS FOR BACK PAIN

- infection (discitis; vertebral osteomyelitis; paraspinal abscess) particularly in obese or diabetic patients
- tumour (metastatic and myeloma)

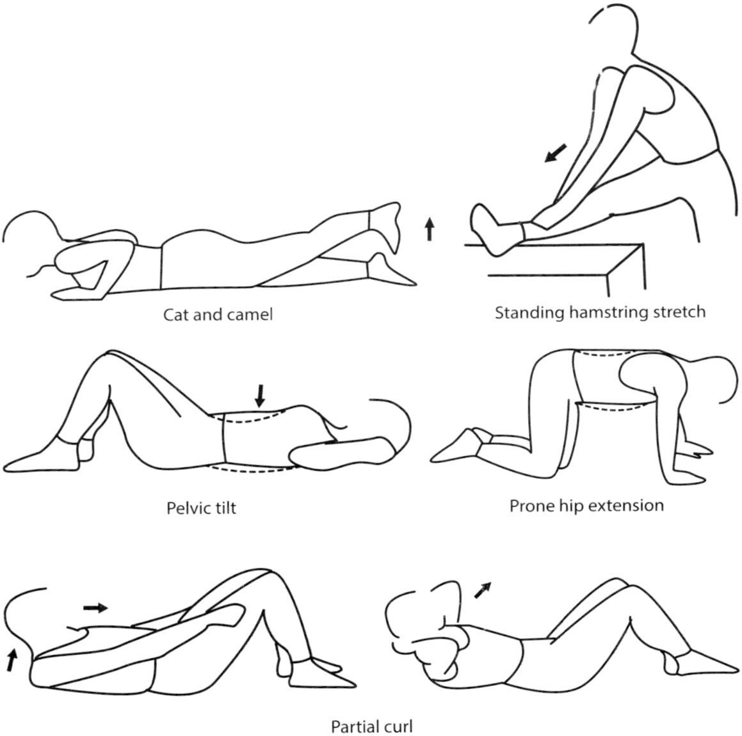

Cat and camel

Standing hamstring stretch

Pelvic tilt

Prone hip extension

Partial curl

Figure 23.4 Back pain prevention exercise regime

- trauma (osteoporotic fractures)
- viscogenic (retroperotoneal mass)

This group of patients should have complete blood work, plain X-rays, and a CT scan of the L-spine, plus possibly a bone scan and MRI, depending on the pathology.

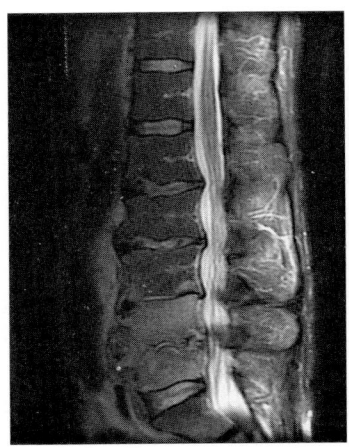

Figure 23.5 MRI of spinal infection

LEG PAIN DOMINANT (SCIATICA)

A smaller group of patients presents to the office with dramatic leg pain. These people are really in distress and do not get better as quickly as lumbago patients. Typically, the pain develops suddenly after an awkward twist of the lower spine or a lift with poor spinal posture. The pain is primarily down one leg to the knee or beyond, is a burning sensation, and is made worse by coughing or straining. These people can barely walk and often crawl around the house to avoid extending their spines.

Neurologic findings may include foot numbness, foot drop of various degrees, loss of ankle reflexes, and positive nerve tension tests. Bowel and bladder patterns may also change, usually because of high analgesic use. True fecal incontinence with poor sphincter tone is rare, but if present, is worrisome for a possible cauda equina syndrome.

Initial treatment should be conservative, including NSAID, rest, local modalities, and then physiotherapy.

Plain X-rays and a CT (or MRI) of the lumbar spine are indicated. The pathology is usually at the L5/S1 > L4/L5 disc space.

Generally, these patients improve over a few weeks (not days, as in mechanical back pain). Probably more than 90% of initial attacks can be treated conservatively. The relative indications for surgery — lumbar discectomy/decompression — are somewhat controversial.[4]

CHECKLIST OF INDICATIONS FOR LUMBAR DISC SURGERY

Absolute

- progressive neurologic deficit (cauda equina syndrome)
- nerve root compression from infection or tumour (rare)

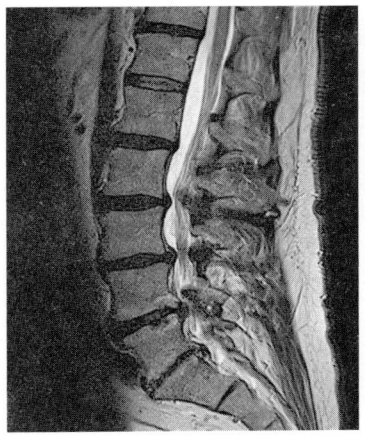 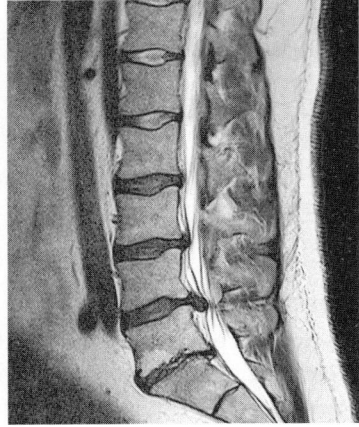

Figure 23.6 MRI showing multilevel lower lumbar spinal stenosis

Figure 23.7 MRI of lumbar disc herniation

Relative

- a surgical lesion: disc/stenotic canal present on CT/MRI in addition to one or more of the following three symptoms:
    - · complete foot drop; no improvement after 2–3 weeks
    - · intractable leg pain; no improvement after 2–3 weeks
    - · recurrent symptoms/severe; with lateral canal stenosis

REFERENCES

1. Shan L, Shan B, Graham D, et al. Total hip replacement: a systematic review and meta-analysis on mid-term quality of life. *Osteoarthritis Cartilage.* 2014;22(3):389–406.

2. Hall H, McIntosh BHK, Melles T. A different approach to back pain diagnosis: identifying a pattern of pain. *Can J Contin Med Educ.* 1994;Feb:31–42.

3. Hall H. Can you spare 10 minutes a day? The New Back Doctor; 1994. p. 183.

4. Loupasis GA, Stamos K, Katonis PG, et al. Seven- to 20-year outcome of lumbar discectomy. *Spine.* 1999;24(22):2313–7. http://dx.doi.org/10.1097/00007632-199911150-00005. Medline:10586454

24

Foot and Ankle

The foot and ankle are common sites of disorders. Most problems occur in the forefoot (great toe > lesser toes) and around the ankle joint and heel.

Forefoot Disorders

The great toe is the keystone to the forefoot: if the great toe is out of alignment, then the whole forefoot is out of balance. Correct the great toe, and most lesser toe problems improve.

HALLUX VALGUS (BUNIONS)

These are not very exciting problems to deal with, but they are quite common and really quite distressing for patients (90% women). Symptoms include an enlarging, ugly bump on the medial side of the great toe, great toe pain at the end of the day, and problems wearing anything but flat, wide shoes.

Once surgery is deemed necessary, patients must be warned that bunion surgery is not a quick fix. They will have pain and swelling for a full 3 months after surgery. The foot will be better, but not normal. There are three typical groups of bunion patients, as outlined in the following checklist.

CHECKLIST OF HALLUX VALGUS PATIENTS

Typical, familial
- middle-aged women
- mild to moderate deformities (< 30 degrees valgus at MTP joint)
- correctible passively to neutral
- congruent MTP joint
- no O/A
- surgery = distal bony procedure (often done by podiatrists)

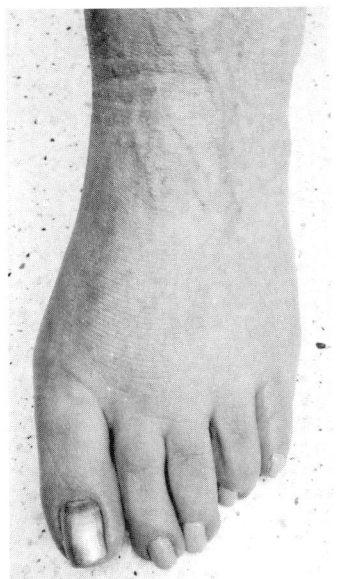

Figure 24.1 Mild to moderate (typical) hallux valgus

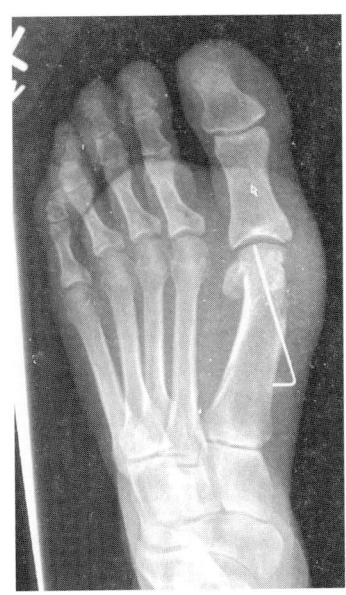

Figure 24.2 Chevron osteotomy

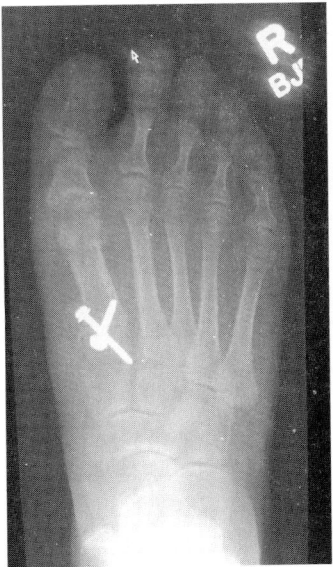

Figure 24.3 PMTO and DSTR for severe adolescent bunions

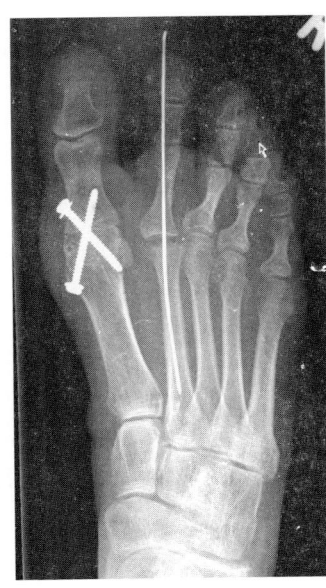

Figure 24.4 Great toe MTP joint fusion and D2 MTP resection and pinning

Adolescent, hypermobile

- hallux valgus > 45 degrees
- very springy deformities
- zigzag feet with metatarsus primus varus
- joint noncongruent
- high recurrence rate
- needs aggressive, proximal repair/osteotomy

Neuromuscular and rheumatoid

- very rigid deformities
- no passive correction
- lesser toes also usually involved
- joint noncongruent/arthritic
- surgery must be aggressive = MTP fusion/lesser toe releases

---

HALLUX RIGIDUS

This disorder can be confused with hallux valgus, but although the great toe is swollen, it is not deviated into valgus. In addition, the hallmark of the diagnosis is stiffness of the great toe MTP joint (particularly for dorsiflexion). This disorder is common in both men and women and often seen in long-distance runners.

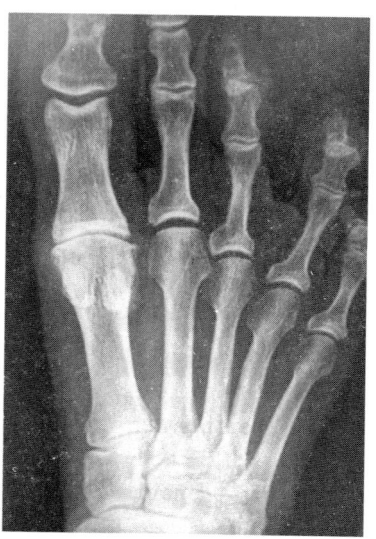

SURGICAL TREATMENT

- if early and joint motion fair–good = cheilectomy (removal of joint spurs)
- if joint mostly destroyed and motion poor = MTP fusion

Figure 24.5 Osteoarthritis of great toe MTP joint (hallux rigidus)

Good pain relief is typical; patients can walk well, but not run, after a fusion.

LESSER TOE DEFORMITIES

Lesser toe deformities are common, but certainly not very glamorous, and are seen in older women in particular. The lesser toes be-

come clawed and twisted, and
the skin between the toes wears
down.

Look for causes of neuro-
muscular imbalance, rheu-
matoid arthritis, or vascular
compromise. Avoid surgery, if
possible (use toe spacers, foot
soaking, and minor footwear
modifications). Podiatrists have
a real role to play here.

If surgery is needed, aggressively release the soft tissues
and fuse the proximal interpha-
langeal (PIP) joints.

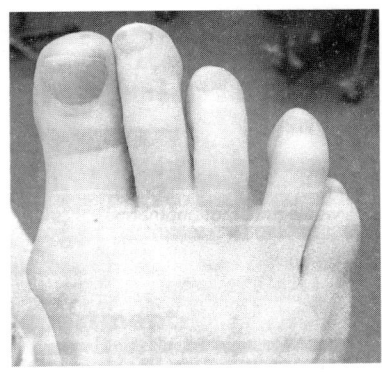

*Figure 24.6 Moderate D3, D4, and D5 claw
toe deformities*

Hind-foot Disorders

HEEL PAIN (PLANTAR FASCIITIS)

Plantar fasciitis is a relatively common problem, in middle-aged
women in particular. One or both heels are exquisitely painful, particularly with the first few steps in the morning. Generally, there is no
history of trauma to the heel.

The physical exam shows normal ankle and hind-foot motion but
point tenderness to deep palpation over the calcaneus and medial
plantar arch. X-rays are normal or may show a small anterior calcaneal bone spur, which is not pathological.

Treatment is conservative: 5% NSAID gels, footwear changes, and
advice never to go barefoot. Surgery is controversial. Most problems
resolve but can take 2–3 years to run their course.

HIND-FOOT STIFFNESS

Hind-foot problems usually involve the ankle joint. Most are the result of ankle or Pilon fractures in the past. The diagnosis is usually
straightforward: the ankle is stiff and swells with walking. A high-energy ankle or Pilon fracture can produce significant ankle osteoarthritis within 2 years; lower-energy fractures take 10–15 years to develop
osteoarthritis.

Surgical treatment in the early stages involves arthroscopy, debridement, or fracture fixation metal removal. For end-stage ankle arthri-

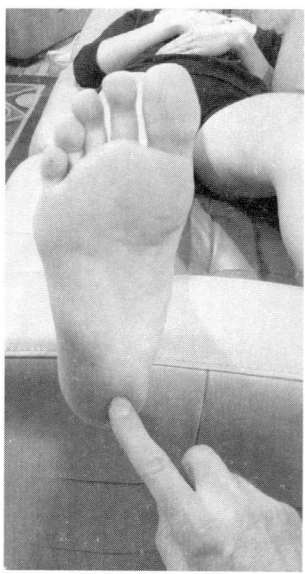

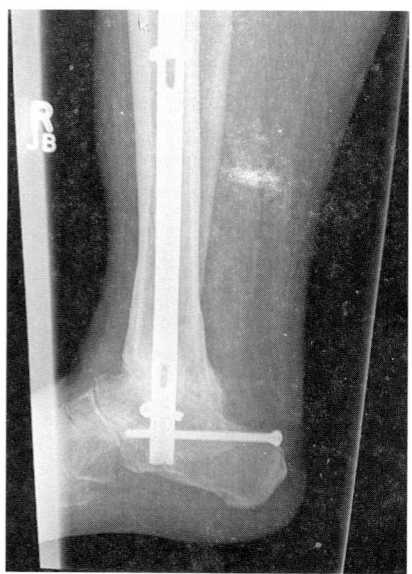

Figure 24.7 Photo demonstrating local tenderness to deep palpation in fasciitis

Figure 24.8 Ankle joint fusion for severe hind-foot arthritis (subtalar joint also fused in this case)

tis, ankle fusion is still the gold standard of surgical treatment. Ankle replacements are possible, but still controversial.

Calcaneal fractures can cause post-traumatic arthritis of the subtalar joint. These patients have problems with walking on uneven ground or slopes though their ankle motion remains good. These patients can be complicated, and many are workers' compensation cases.

Surgical options include subtalar joint fusion once conservative modalities have been exhausted.

RHEUMATOID ARTHRITIS

These patients usually have forefoot involvement, but sometimes quite severe hind-foot involvement as well. Quite horrendous valgus deformities can occur. Surgery must be aggressive and requires the fusion of any joint involved.

25

Hand, Wrist, and Elbow

Hand and Wrist Disorders

Wrist and hand disorders are less commonly seen in the office. Many symptoms are intermittent and mild so people tend to live with them, preferring to get their knees and shoulders fixed first (particularly rheumatoid patients).

CARPAL TUNNEL SYNDROME

Mild carpal tunnel syndrome is quite common in older patients with arthritis in their hands, in diabetics, and in patients prone to swelling. Typically, there is pain and numbness in the thumb and index/long fingers, which is worse at night and with repetitive use of the hand.

If symptoms are intermittent, treatment is NSAID and extension night splints. If numbness is progressive, or constant, then surgical release is advised. Nerve conduction tests should confirm preoperative diagnosis. Look for thenar

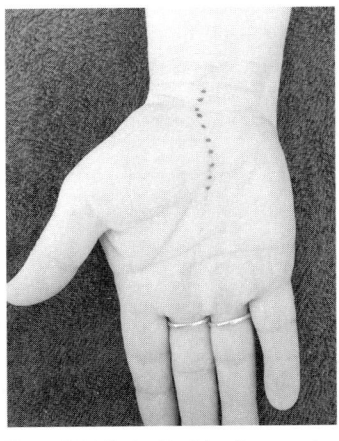

Figure 25.1 Typical incision for carpal tunnel release

muscle atrophy that, if present, is suggestive of severe medial nerve entrapment.

THUMB PAIN

The thumb is frequently painful because of osteoarthritis at the carpal-metacarpal (CMC) joint (particularly in older women) and at the metacarpal phalangeal (MP) joint in rheumatoid arthritis. Thumb opposition and pinch grip can be severely limited.

Treatment begins with hand NSAID gels and splints. If changes are progressive, the patient can be referred to a hand/wrist surgeon. The CMC joint can be decompressed with a tendon interposition and the rheumatoid MP joint can be replaced.

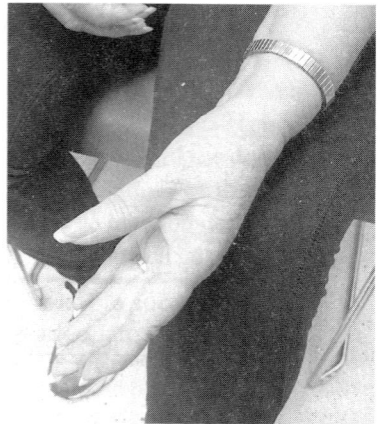

Figure 25.2 O/A of thumb CMC joint

TENDONOPATHIES OF THE FINGERS AND THUMB

Patients can develop stenosing tenosynovitis (trigger finger) of the thumb at the first extensor wrist compartment (de Quervain's) on the extensor side of the hand or of any finger flexor tendon at the CMC joint level in the palm. On the flexor side of the hand, any of the long flexor tendons of the fingers or the thumb may develop stenosing tenosynovitis at the MP joint level, in the palm where the tendon pulleys catch on the thickened flexor tendons.

Look for catching/locking of the finger and a painful swelling over the constriction. Surgical release of the tendon sheath is curative for both conditions.

WRIST STIFFNESS

RHEUMATOID ARTHRITIS

Rheumatoid arthritis can severely affect the hand and wrist with both tenosynovitis and bony destruction of joints. The pattern of collapse/supination of the wrist and ulnar deviation/deformities of the fingers is classic, so diagnosis is never difficult. Amazingly, these patients seem to carry on for years with hand/wrist deformities and choose instead to have their lower limbs dealt

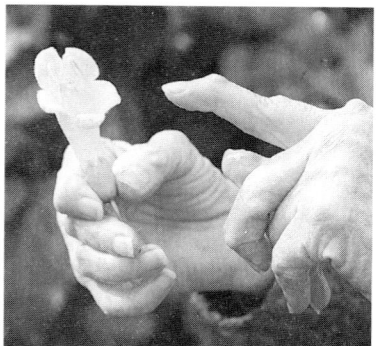

Figure 25.3 Advanced rheumatoid hand and wrist deformities

with first. Custom splinting helps. Watch for possible extensor tendon rupture if tenosynovitis becomes severe.

Rheumatoid hand and wrist reconstruction is possible at several joint levels (partial or complete fusions of the wrist or replacements/ balancing of the finger joints). These patients should be referred to a surgeon specializing in the rheumatoid hand and to a team of therapists for rehabilitation postoperatively.

OSTEOARTHRITIS

Osteoarthritic patients present classically with an acute on chronic history of dorsal wrist pain and swelling. The wrist was always a little weak, and then it really bothered them after a recent fall or sprain. Typically, these are middle-aged men with a history of heavy wrist abuse and trauma (e.g., rodeo riders).

The physical exam shows chronic swelling and pain over the dorsal radial wrist, decreased dorsiflexion, and often supination.

Plain X-rays clinch the diagnosis. There are four patterns (listed in order of frequency seen):

1. scaphoid fracture nonunion (with collapse = SNAC wrist)
2. scapholunate ligament, old injury with collapse = SLAC wrist
3. old intra-articular wrist fracture with radial/carpal O/A
4. AVN lunate (Kienboch's disease)

Most of these patients are not keen on surgery and do well with splints and NSAIDs initially. A *staged approach* to surgery can follow to try to maintain as much wrist ROM for as long as possible:

- wrist arthroscopy
- open debridements
- partial wrist fusions (to unload the arthritic areas)
- full radiocarpal (wrist) fusions

Wrist replacement arthroplasty is not generally an option for the osteoarthritic wrist.[1]

WRIST MECHANICAL PROBLEMS

This group of patients presents with primarily movement-related wrist problems, usually after a recent injury. There are two groups: (a) those with wrist fracture malunion/radial wrist pain/stiffness and (b) those with ulnar wrist pain/supination problems.

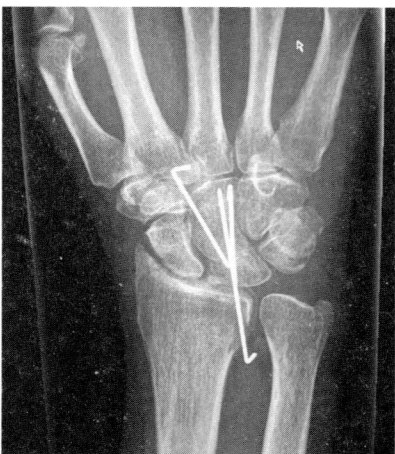

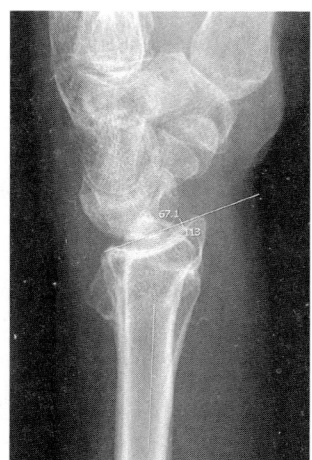

Figure 25.4 Partial carpal fusion using K-wires

Figure 25.5 Wrist fracture malunion (Note radial shortening and abnormal dorsal tilting of joint.)

WRIST FRACTURE MALUNION/RADIAL WRIST PAIN/STIFFNESS

These patients have had a distal radius fracture that has healed with some deformity (usually dorsal tilting and shortening; volar tilting is less common but tolerated less well by patients). Joint space is usually okay, but cosmetically the patient does not like the wrist's appearance. The wrist aches with use, and there is loss of supination and higher degrees of palmar and dorsiflexion.

Treatment includes extra-articular osteotomy of the radius (to correct sagittal deformity and shortening).

ULNAR WRIST PAIN/SUPINATION PROBLEMS

These involve disorders of the cartilage at the distal end of the ulna (distal radial ulnar joint or DRUJ). These disorders are typically seen in young women who have slender, hypermobile wrist joints. The hallmark of the diagnosis is sharp, catching, dorsal ulnar-sided wrist pain with wrist rotation (particularly supination), local distal ulna tenderness, and laxity of the DRUJ on provocative testing.

X-rays may show an old radius fracture with mild shortening and impaction of the distal ulna, or the ulna may be naturally a little longer than the radius. An MRI may be helpful to document a TFCC tear (triangular fibrocartilage complex).

If wrist splinting fails, surgical options include the following:
- wrist arthroscopic debridement
- open DRUJ repair
- ulnar shortening

Elbow Disorders

The elbow is a common site of intermittent, mild problems but it is not a commonly operated upon joint. Any decision to operate around the elbow should be tempered with the knowledge that the elbow, more than any other joint, *gets stiff* after immobilization and surgery.

TENNIS ELBOW SYNDROME

Tennis elbow is a common, generally self-limited disorder seen in middle-aged adults who do repetitive work with the upper extremities; many are workers' compensation cases.

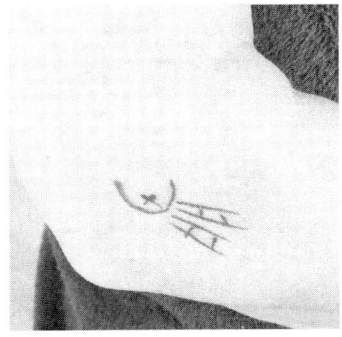

Look for point tenderness over the lateral humeral epicondyle. X-rays and nerve conduction studies (NCS) are generally normal.

Figure 25.6 Tennis elbow muscle insertion point

Treatment is *95% non-surgical* and includes NSAID, gels, a forearm strap, physiotherapy, and local Depo-Medrol injections (< 2 per year). For the 5% who require *surgical* treatment, arthroscopic or open release is used but results are variable.[2] Most improve (burn out) spontaneously after 2–3 years; hopefully the patient's modified work program lasts as long.

OLECRANON BURSITIS

Bursitis is a common problem for older men who constantly bump their elbows (truck drivers, farmers). The tip of the olecranon becomes reddened and, sometimes, hugely swollen. Elbow motion always remains good since the elbow joint itself is not involved. An elbow X-ray shows normal anatomy or may reveal a small posterior olecranon spur.

Treatment is conservative unless the bursa starts to drain and becomes secondarily infected, requiring a radical bursectomy down

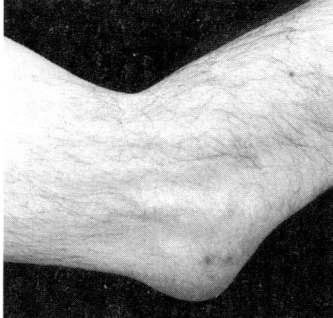

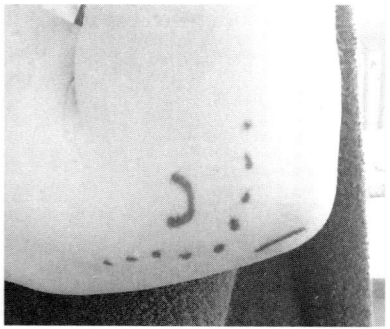

Figure 25.7 Olecranon bursitis

Figure 25.8 Outline of ulnar nerve at cubital tunnel at elbow

to the bone. Expect the sac to fill with blood postoperatively and require aspiration. Ultimately, recovery is uncomplicated.

ULNAR NERVE ENTRAPMENT (CUBITAL TUNNEL SYNDROME)

This uncommon disorder is usually seen in older patients who present with pain and numbness in their ulnar (fourth and fifth fingers). The patient has a clumsy handgrip and small hand muscle wasting. They often present quite late.

- Local tenderness and swelling is typical. NCS confirms the diagnosis.
- Surgical release +/– transposition of ulnar nerve = treatment
- Results are variable and prognosis is guarded since patients often present so late, especially if muscle atrophy is present pre-operatively.

ELBOW STIFFNESS

As noted, elbow stiffness can be a real problem with any trauma around the elbow. There are a few common subtypes:

INTERMITTENT; LOOSE BODIES

Young adults can present with intermittent symptoms of elbow locking and pain. Often, there has been a long history of these events and a distant, relatively minor injury. X-rays show normal anatomy or may show loose ossified bodies or OCD. Treatment is arthroscopic or open loose body removal.

PROGRESSIVE; NON-RHEUMATOID

This is the more common pattern. Patients have a distant injury and with every new strain, the elbow does not fully recover but gets stiffer.

The stiffness arises from soft tissue contractures around the elbow joint and from joint incongruity within the joint.

X-rays show one of three patterns:

- mild joint O/A with heterotopic bone formation
- moderate ulna/humeral joint O/A
- severe global elbow O/A

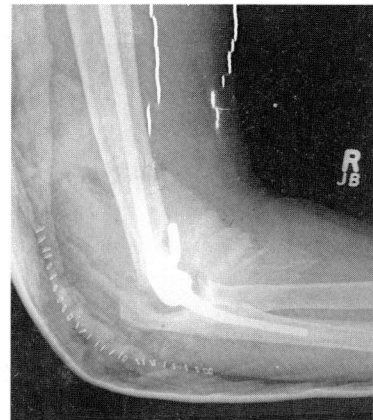

Figure 25.9 Total elbow replacement

The only good thing about elbow stiffness is that one does not need much elbow motion to be "functional" in ADL. If up to 180 degrees is the normal range of motion, the functional range is between 30–95 degrees. Pronation/Supination should also be > 45 degrees in each direction.

Surgery should be deferred until the patient is approaching the functional ROM and is then done on a graduated basis (similar to wrist reconstruction):

- arthroscopic debridement/releases
- open releases/interpositions
- arthroplasties (partial or total elbow)
- fusion

All these elbow procedures are quite technically demanding, so referral to a dedicated elbow surgeon is usually recommended.

RHEUMATOID

Rheumatoid patients have a lot of trouble with their elbows but, as with their wrists, rarely request surgery until their lower limb problems are treated first. As in the wrist, there is a gradual progression of involvement around the elbow from rheumatoid nodules, to synovitis with intact joint surfaces, to isolated radiocapitellar involvement, to global joint loss and bone erosion.

A stepwise approach should be taken with these patients (medically and surgically) depending on what part of the elbow is involved. Surgical procedures include open synovectomies and nodule excisions, radiocapitellar joint arthroplasties, and total joint replacements.

Total elbow replacements do well in rheumatoid patients, but they have a high postoperative complication rate[3] (ulnar nerve, wound healing, etc.) and should generally be done by an experienced elbow surgeon.

REFERENCES

1. Weiss KE, Rodner CM. Osteoarthritis of the wrist. *J Hand Surg Am*. 2007;32(5):725–46. http://dx.doi.org/10.1016/j.jhsa.2007.02.003. Medline:17482013

2. Boyer MI, Hastings II H. Lateral tennis elbow: "Is there any science out there?" *J Shoulder Elbow Surg*. 1999;8(5):481–91. http://dx.doi.org/10.1016/S1058-2746(99)90081-2. Medline:10543604

3. Little CP, Graham AJ, Karatzas G, et al. Outcomes of total elbow arthroplasty for rheumatoid arthritis: comparative study of three implants. *J Bone Joint Surg Am*. 2005;87(11):2439–48. http://dx.doi.org/10.2106/JBJS.D.02927. Medline:16264119

PART FIVE

ELECTIVE ORTHOPAEDICS IN CHILDREN

26

Infants and Toddlers

This chapter will focus on the common and important topics one will see in community orthopaedic practice with infants and young children. We will limit the discussion to otherwise healthy children. A whole discipline of orthopaedic surgery deals with the various MSK problems that children with muscle and nerve imbalance develop from congenital or developmental syndromes. These are very important in that small population of children but are beyond the scope of this text.

Developmental Dysplasia of the Hip (DDH)

Hip dysplasia is a very important topic for primary-care physicians and orthopaedic surgeons, as the condition is completely preventable, is still relatively common, and has serious consequences if missed. The risk factors are well known and well described:

- prematurity
- breech presentation
- female babies
- floppy babies
- torticollis
- positive family history

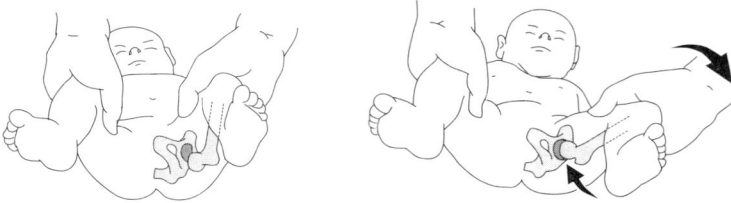

Figure 26.1 Ortolani test: Try to rereduce the hip by lifting anteriorly.

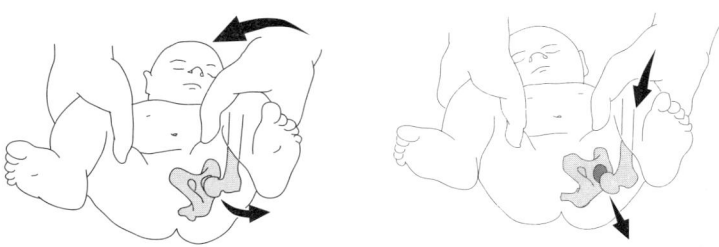

Figure 26.2 Barlow's test: Try to dislocate the hip posteriorly.

Diagnosis is clinical and takes some practice. The Ortolani abduction test and the Barlow posterior subluxation test should be familiar to all family doctors. The tests should be repeated as often as is necessary to monitor the stability of the hip. Any hip that feels unstable should be splinted in abduction and flexion and followed closely both clinically and radiographically.

Hip ultrasound has become a safe and sensitive serial test to follow at-risk hips. Plain AP pelvis radiographs will show more advanced abnormalities, particularly after the newborn stage.

There are standard measurements in the orthopaedic literature that we use to determine if the acetabulum is forming properly and whether the femoral head is centred in the hip joint or moving superiorly:

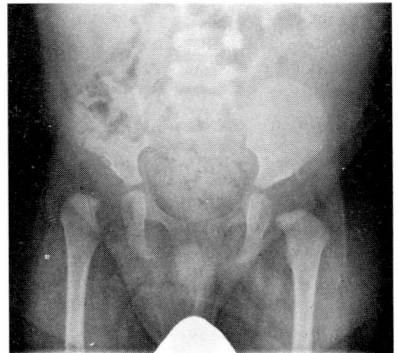

Figure 26.3 AP pelvis X-ray demonstrating right-sided DDH features in a 6-month-old child

- Shenton's line (smooth or broken?)

- acetabular index (should be less than 25 degrees by 6 months)
- centre edge angle (should be 10 degrees or greater)

The treatment of the hip at risk depends primarily on the age at original diagnosis, as outlined in the following checklist.

CHECKLIST FOR DDH BY AGE OF DIAGNOSIS

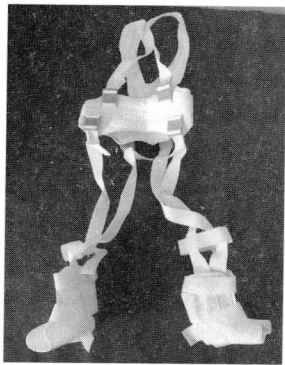

Figure 26.4 Pavlik harness: keeps hips in safe (abducted) position

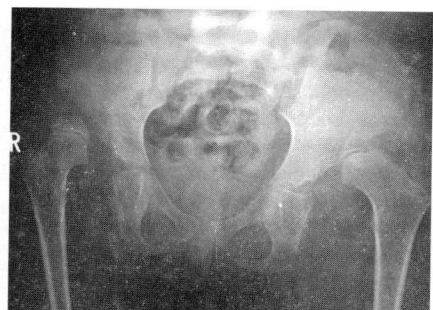

Figure 26.5 Late presentation of bilateral hip dislocations in an older child

0 to 6 months

- most cases, the later the diagnosis, the longer the time in a brace
- use abduction harness of choice (Pavlik, etc.) until hip is stable clinically and X-ray parameters are improving (months)
- wean to splints over several weeks
- patient should be followed by paediatric orthopaedic group

6 to 12 months

- look for asymmetrical hip creases and lack of hip abduction
- abnormal pelvic X-ray
- direct referral to paediatric orthopaedic centre needed
- use tendon releases and serial hip spica casting
- serious, long-term follow-up needed

Older than 12 months (after walking)

- look for a painless limp, a classic sign of DDH
- lack of hip abduction
- leg length shortening
- very serious: hip may not ever be normal
- urgent referral to paediatric orthopaedic surgeon
- use tendon releases and casting, if early
- requires pelvic osteotomies, if late (Salter, etc.)

If diagnosed and treated in the first two age groups, hips with dysplasia have a good prognosis. However, the last group of children (older than 12 months of age at diagnosis) has a more guarded prognosis. The child will usually limp and have leg length discrepancies and weakness in the legs. If they are fortunate, patients will not develop AVN of the femoral head. Inevitably, osteoarthritis of the hip joint will develop if the condition presents after walking age and if the joint is not perfectly reduced in the acetabulum. The age that arthritic symptoms present varies widely, but most DDH patients will seek orthopaedic consultation in their twenties.

Orthopaedic specialists try to defer the age of hip replacement as long as possible because the failure rate is so high in these otherwise healthy, young, active patients.[1] Unfortunately, there are no other surgical options and the surgeon and patient must balance the risk of long-term loosening with short-term quality-of-life benefits.

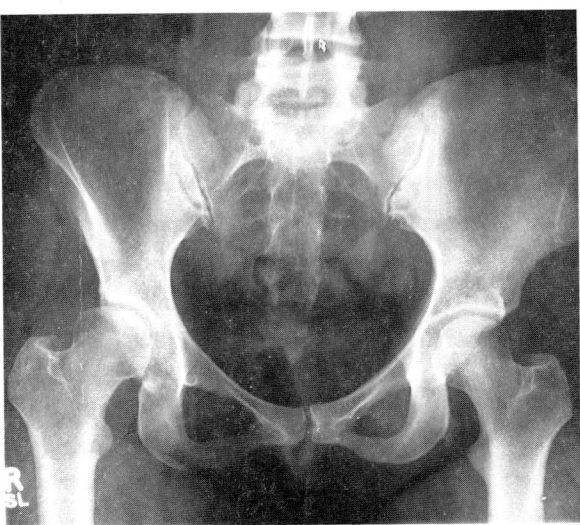

Figure 26.6 Right hip dysplasia in an adult (Right femoral head is uncovered by steep acetabulum.)

Crooked Feet

Children's foot problems are common. Most, but not all, are positional and will improve with age. The key factor is in determining how rigid the deformity is. The more passively correctable, the better. There are two major types of crooked feet: varus and valgus.

Varus Foot

Varus foot includes the "clubfoot deformity" and its variants.

CLUBFOOT

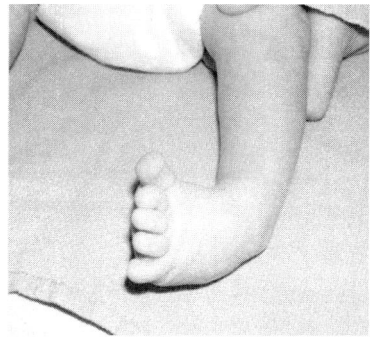

Figure 26.7 Severe left clubfoot deformity

- also known as talipes equino varus (TEV)
- may be unilateral or bilateral
- appears in boys more than girls
- may be a positive family history
- associated with prematurity
- idiopathic (flexible) versus teratogenic (rigid)
- treatment: serial casting (should be done by an experienced orthopaediatric team)

The Ponseti technique of serial casting has been popularized in the past decade. It has decreased the failure rate of casting and the need for corrective surgery.[2]

These patients need to be followed closely because some feet will not fully correct even with serial casting. If they do not correct, surgical release by a paediatric orthopaedic surgeon will be required, usually before the age of 6 months, followed by more serial casting. Treatment involves a tremendous commitment on the part of the parents for the first year or two of the child's life. The most rigid feet will often need repeat surgery as the foot grows, and these feet will never be completely normal. Again, the best predictor of outcome is how rigid the foot was at the outset.

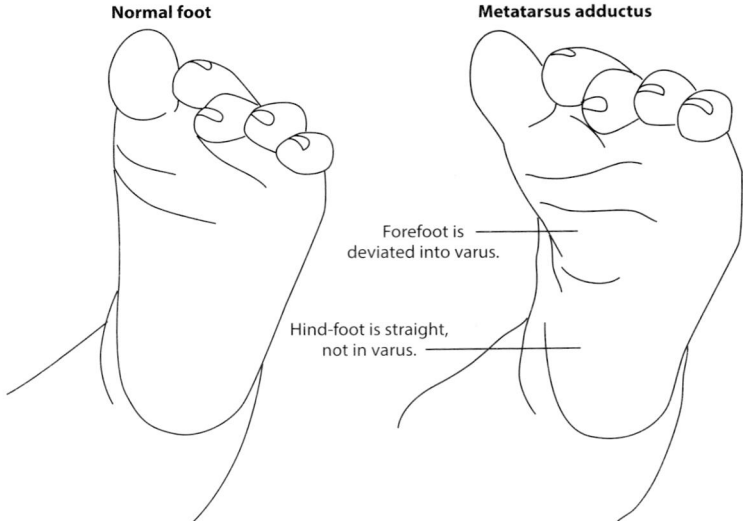

Figure 26.8 Metatarsus adductus: X-rays are normal, other than varus of the forefoot.

METATARSUS ADDUCTUS

Metatarsus adductus is a milder condition than TEV, is easier to treat, and does not involve the hind-foot. This is the key to the diagnosis: the hind-foot is not in varus!

Treatment is always nonsurgical but involves long periods of stretching the muscles and reverse last shoes. Tight feet may require serial casting, but the disorder does not cause lifelong foot problems.

Valgus Foot

The key question to ask in the diagnosis of the valgus foot is, "How flexible is the deformity?" The more rigid it is, the worse it is, just as in the varus foot.

FLEXIBLE VALGUS FOOT

This is a common condition, often bilateral, and is seen in infants with decreased muscle tone and young children with flexible joints. X-rays of the feet are normal apart from a flat plantar arch.

Treatment is conservative and includes stretching techniques, serial casting if the foot is resistant, and good supportive shoes after walking age.

The tendency toward flat feet and weak ankles will persist in some of these children throughout their lifetime.

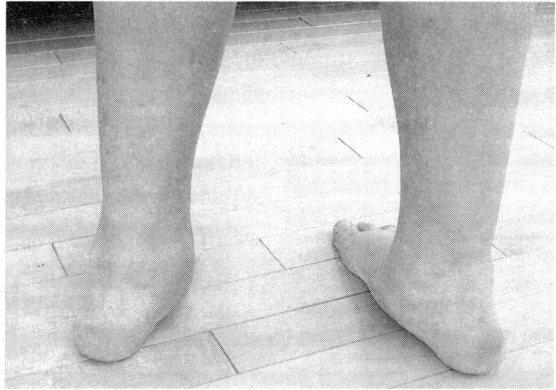

Figure 26.9 Photo of a valgus foot (Most deformities are flexible.)

RIGID VALGUS FOOT

The rigid valgus foot is uncommon and usually unilateral, but can be serious. The hind-foot does not passively correct to neutral. There are two major groups: (a) congenital vertical talus (CVT), a rare condition seen in very young children, and (b) spastic peroneal flatfoot (SPF) valgus seen in older children, caused by a painful lesion in the hind-foot, such as an infection, tumour, or bony bridge.

X-rays, CT scan, and MRI will all show abnormalities. Treatment deals with removing the underlying cause, often surgically.

Gait Problems

Children are often brought into the office by their parents (or grand-parents) with gait problems. The three types seen are in-toers, out-to-ers, and tiptoe gait. The topic of the limping child (painful or painless) was dealt with in detail in Chapter 3 and will not be rediscussed here.

Diagnostic questions include the following:

- Is the child otherwise healthy, or is this a manifestation of an underlying muscle imbalance problem (such as mild cerebral palsy or early muscular dystrophy)?
- Is the problem bilateral and symmetrical or unilateral and unbalanced? Pathological conditions are much more likely to be unilateral and asymmetrical.

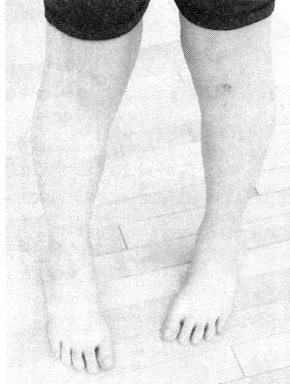 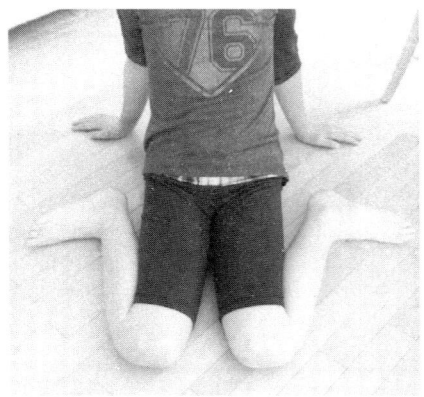

Figure 26.10 Typical gait for in-toeing

Figure 26.11 Comfortable sitting position for in-toers (W-position)

In-toers

These children look pigeon-toed but not awkward; they are active and usually good runners. The toes turn in more when they are tired at the end of day. The problem is usually bilateral and symmetrical. Check the rotational profile of the hip, tibia, and foot as all are involved to some degree.

Treatment for in-toeing is as follows:

- Rule out any underlying causes and then reassure parents.
- stretching exercises
- good-quality shoes (not custom)
- will improve over time; some may persist into adulthood to some degree
- avoid the W-position (It is amazing how many of these children find this sitting position comfortable!)

Out-toers (Knock-kneed)

Out-toers have flexible joints in general, move slower, and look more awkward than the in-toer group. Many of these children tend to be overweight and have valgus, hyperextendable knees and flexible, flat, valgus feet.

Check for asymmetry and any underlying disorders; then treatment is conservative, including good supportive shoes and weight loss. These children, especially girls, can develop problems with lateral patellar dislocations, later in their teenage years, due to their patellar

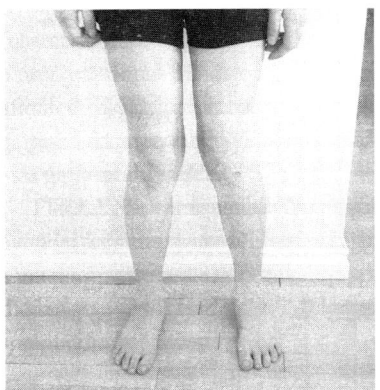

Figure 26.12 Bilateral genu valgum; common in out-toer type gait

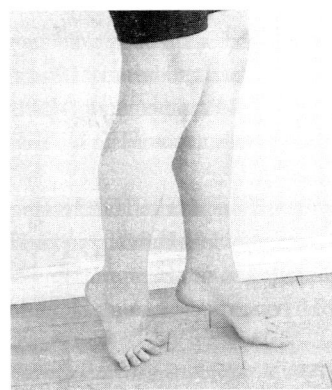

Figure 26.13 Tiptoe gait; symmetrical type

malalignment. Weight loss and good leg muscle fitness are the best preventative measures.

This alignment pattern can produce chronic painful flat feet in adulthood, which does not produce arthritis but can be quite disabling.

Tiptoe Gait

This condition is common in children with neuromuscular imbalance (such as mild cerebral palsy), but it is uncommon in otherwise healthy children. We often see this temporarily in healthy children after a cast has been removed, especially when the child is tired, but it resolves spontaneously after a few weeks.

If any underlying cause has been ruled out, and if the gait is symmetrical, then the problem is most likely habitual, or idiopathic, and treatment should begin, starting with stretching and physiotherapy. Refer the patient to a paediatric orthopaedic centre if this fails. They may add serial casting. Surgical Achilles tendon releases are reserved for resistant cases.

REFERENCES

1. Dudkiewicz I, Salai M, Ganel A, et al. Total hip arthroplasty in patients younger than 30 years of age following developmental dysplasia of hip (DDH) in infancy. *Arch Orthop Trauma Surg.* 2002;122(3):139–42. http://dx.doi.org/10.1007/s004020100307. Medline:11927994

2. Herzenberg JE, Radler C, Bor N. Ponseti versus traditional methods of casting for idiopathic clubfoot. *J Pediatr Orthop.* 2002;22(4):517–21. http://dx.doi.org/10.1097/01241398-200207000-00019. Medline:12131451

27

Adolescents and Teenagers

Adolescents and teenagers are not frequently seen in the office for elective conditions; however, three important conditions may arise in this age group: (a) scoliosis, (b) overuse syndromes, and (c) back and limb pain.

Scoliosis

Scoliosis, especially idiopathic scoliosis, is an important topic in primary care since these adolescent girls usually first present to their family doctors. The remaining two classes of scoliosis (congenital and neuromuscular) usually present at much earlier ages to paediatricians who are already involved in the care of these children.

The largest group, *idiopathic*, develops in otherwise healthy children, usually girls, for no apparent reason, but seems to be decreasing in prevalence in North America in the last decade. Look for a positive family history and often a tall, slim build.

Screening protocols exist for adolescent girls[1] but are not widely followed. Regardless, a clinical screening "forward bend-over test" is simple and should be done for girls aged 11–15 years. X-rays are only needed if abnormalities are discovered. If ordered, they should be standing thoracolumbar full-length views.

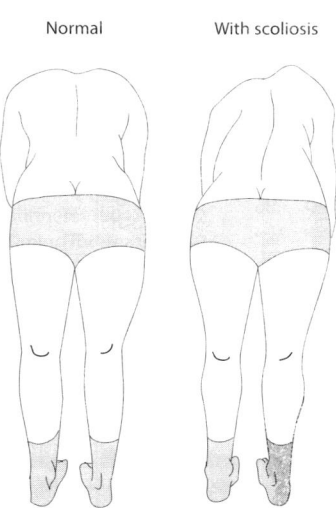

Normal   With scoliosis

Figure 27.1 The diagram on the right shows thoracolumbar curve convex to the right.

CHECKLIST OF PARAMETERS TO CONSIDER
- size of the curve (greater than 15–20 degrees?)
- skeletal maturity (years of growth left?)
- flexibility of curve
- spine balanced?

Worrisome features
- curve greater than 35 degrees
- double curves
- poor spinal balance
- stiff curves
- skeletally immature girl

Treatment
- curve greater than 15–20 degrees → refer to a paediatric scoliosis centre
- moderate curve (> 25–35 degrees) → add back bracing
- severe curve (> 45 degrees with high risk of progression) → add surgery
- regular follow-up to assess progression of the curve
- stretching exercises and physiotherapy

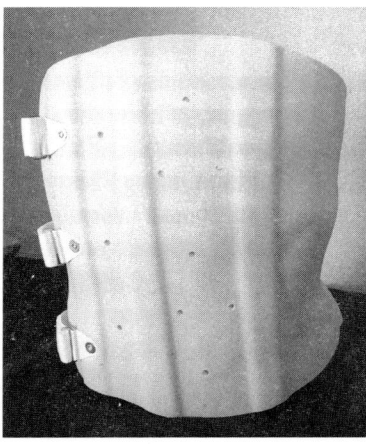

Figure 27.2 Scoliosis Boston Brace

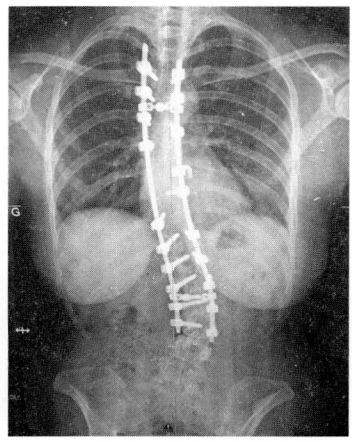

Figure 27.3 Thoracolumbar corrective scoliosis surgery

Scoliosis treatment and surgery is a highly subspecialized area of paediatric orthopaedics. Specialists in this area are regularly revising the parameters for surgery and the techniques used. The previous are, therefore, only general guidelines. Once your patient is enrolled in the scoliosis clinic, they will follow the child for years, until adulthood.

Adolescent Overuse Syndromes

KNEE PAIN: GIRLS

Knee pain is very common in teenage girls and can be so debilitating that they often drop out of all activities. Check for the following:

- pain/tenderness globally situated over the anterior patella
- constant ache after activities
- may be associated with mild swelling
- true locking is unusual
- some may have patellar instability (sublux laterally)
- X-rays and MRI = normal (or valgus alignment)

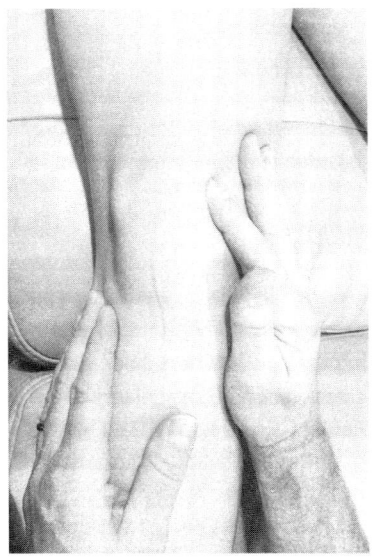

Figure 27.4 Patellar apprehension test (lateral force applied)

This condition is called *chondromalacia patella*. Treatment involves NSAID, physiotherapy, a soft knee brace, and then return to selected sports. In recalcitrant cases, arthroscopic debridement (to smooth undersurface of patella) may be required. Empirically, arthroscopy can be quite effective to break the cycle of pain and anxiety in these selective and resistant cases.

KNEE PAIN: BOYS

Boys can also get diffuse anterior knee pain, but it is much less common than in girls. Boys are much more likely to present with extensor mechanism overuse symptoms related to sports. The usual age is 12–15 years old, before the growth plates fuse. This syndrome covers a spectrum from reversible patellar tendonitis, to tendon thickening, to true tibial tubercle apophysitis (Osgood-Schlatter's disease).

Diagnosis is made by point tenderness, often with swelling over the tibial tubercle and patellar tendon. X-rays may show fragmentation of the tibial tubercle on the lateral view.

Treatment is conservative: NSAID, splinting (or casting) the knee in extension for 3–4 weeks, and limiting jumping sports until the swelling subsides.

Occasionally, adults present with very large and tender tibial tubercles from previous Osgood-Schlatter's disease from which the overgrown bone must be excised. This is almost never done before the apophysis has fused to the tibia.

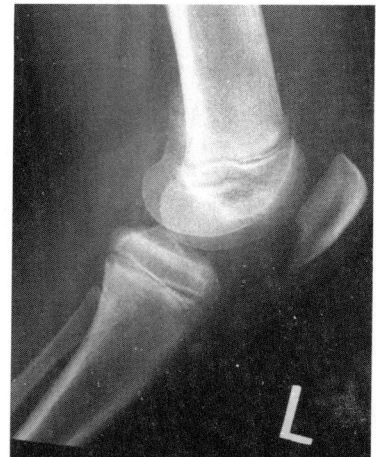

Figure 27.5 Fragmented tibial tubercle on X-ray

ANKLE ROLLERS

Some older children will present with chronically weak ankles, more commonly girls than boys, especially those with lax joints generally. The ankle will roll/invert on rough terrain, or with some sports, and then swell. A history of ankle sprain (inadequately treated) is usual.

The physical exam will reveal the ankle may be lax generally or may show increased translation on varus testing. X-rays appear normal.

Treatment includes an over-the-counter ankle brace and physiotherapy. If the condition is debilitating and asymmetrical, surgery may be done once the growth plates are fused.

AVULSIONS AROUND THE HIP

These are uncommon but dramatic injuries, often seen in athletic girls and boys in the 12- to 17-year age group. While lunging in hockey, track and field, or dancing, a sudden pain is felt in the anterior hip/groin area with an immediate loss of power and the ability even to walk. This history is classic.

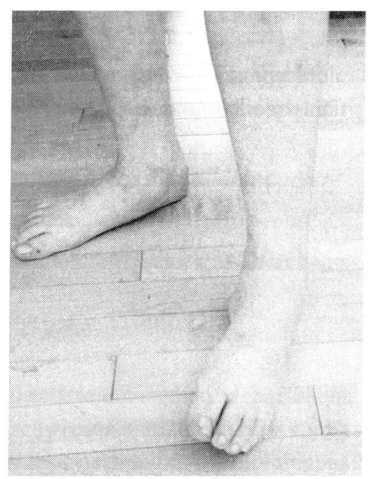

Figure 27.6 Inversion instability of left ankle

X-rays confirm the diagnosis: a bony avulsion of the apophysis at a major muscle attachment. Avulsions can occur at the lesser or greater trochanter of the hip, or the anterior or inferior iliac spine area on the pelvis.

Treatment is supportive: crutches, NSAID for 3–4 weeks, physiotherapy, and no sports for 4–8 weeks. Surgery is rarely needed.

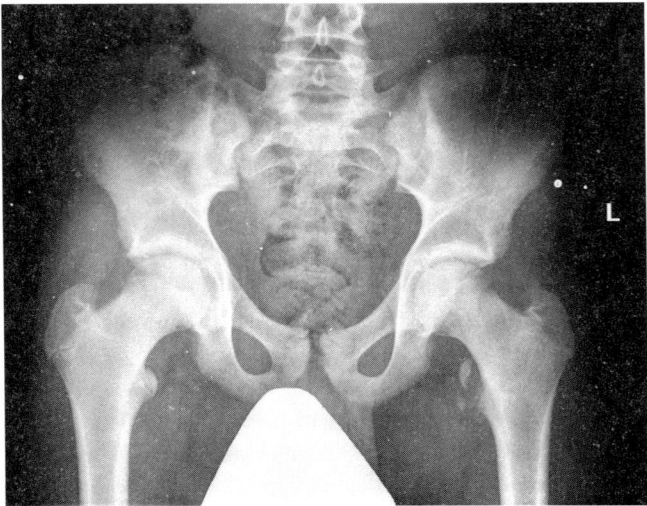

Figure 27.7 Avulsion of the left lesser trochanter of hip

Back and Limb Pain

Chronic back or limb pain is uncommon in otherwise healthy children. A few pathological conditions must be ruled out, but most seem to be manifestations of stress in the child's life. Issues related to school or family disharmony are usually the underlying stressor.

Pathological Back Pain

The following conditions are uncommon, but important to rule out, because they are serious.

CHECKLIST OF DIFFERENTIAL DIAGNOSIS FOR PATHOLOGICAL BACK PAIN

Lumbar spondylolisthesis

- lower lumbar spine; congenital fibrous weak link in posterior spinal arch
- adolescent girls; often gymnasts or dancers; overuse injury
- X-ray = diagnostic
- treatment: time off sports; physiotherapy; brace
- surgical fusion if severe and progressive (uncommon)

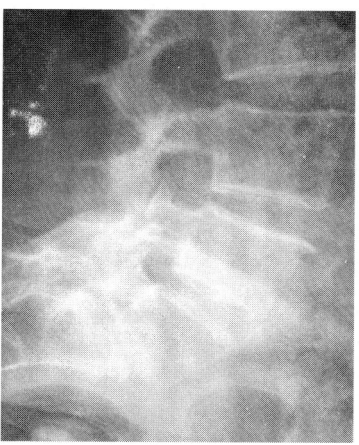 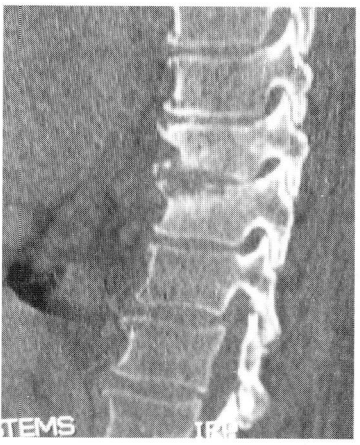

Figure 27.8 Slip of L5 on S1 vertebra (Note the posterior pars defect at L5 level.)

Figure 27.9 Discitis (Note the obvious difference in disc height.)

Spinal infection

- discitis, or osteomyelitis, or both
- severe back pain; very tender and rigid spine locally
- hematogenous: *Staphylococcus aureus* or tuberculosis
- if immunocompromised: any bacteria
- CT/MRI needed to assess bony canal and neural elements
- Treatment: IV antibiotics; brace
- surgery if paraspinal abscess; instability/collapse

Spinal tumours

- rare, but serious
- osteoblastoma (classic spinal tumour of children)
- marrow tumours (leukemia; lymphoma; Ewing's)
- full staging work-up needed
- treatment: varies greatly on tumour type and stage

Pathological Limb Pain

These are uncommon in healthy children but are important to rule out. Children often have systemic symptoms, such as weight loss or fatigue, which are unusual in functional limb pain. There is a wide differential diagnosis, outlined in the following checklist.

CHECKLIST OF DIFFERENTIAL DIAGNOSIS FOR PATHOLOGICAL LIMB PAIN

Inflammatory

JUVENILE RHEUMATOID ARTHRITIS (JRA)

- new term is juvenile idiopathic arthritis (JIA)
- well-described diagnostic criteria exist[2]
- can be episodic, remitting, or progressive and lifelong
- various patterns of joint involvement exist; any joint in the body can be involved
- treatment should be coordinated by a paediatric rheumatologist

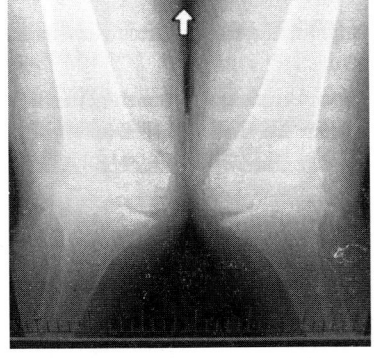

Figure 27.10 Severe valgus knee deformities from longstanding JRA

ANKYLOSING SPONDYLITIS

- teenage boys
- HLA-B27 antigen
- positive family history in males
- spine > hips > knees
- start of lifelong disease? (variable course)

Infection

- hematogenous
- healthy or immunosuppressed children
- various levels of involvement:
  - cellulitis
  - fasciitis
  - osteomyelitis
- septic arthritis
- see Chapter 3 for details of work-up and treatment

Tumours

NONAGGRESSIVE
- unicameral bone cysts
- fibrous dysplasia
- fibrous cortical defects

AGGRESSIVE
- leukemia
- lymphoma
- osteogenic sarcoma
- Ewing's sarcoma

Metabolic/Vascular
- Rickets: crooked painful limbs; rare unless vitamin D deficient
- SCFE = acute on chronic hip pain seen in obese adolescent boys
- Perthes disease: idiopathic avascular necrosis of the femoral head; seen in 8- to 12-year-old children
- hemophilia: rare cause of hemarthrosis and joint destruction in poorly controlled patients only
- renal disease: rare in children; bone cysts and stress fractures
- diabetes: fatigue, joint pains, and tendonopathies

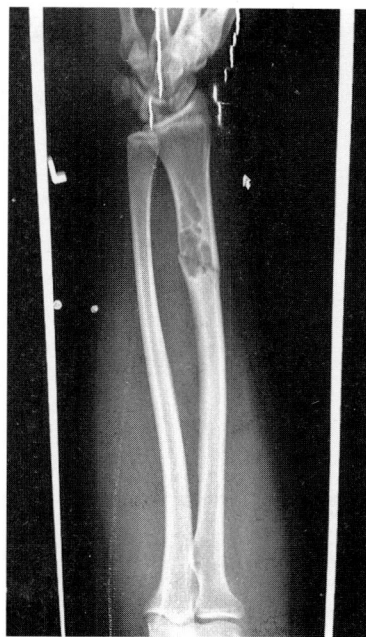

Figure 27.11 Nonaggressive hole in bone with fracture (Note the sharp margins.)

REFERENCES
1. Roubal PJ, Freeman DC, Placzek JD. Costs and effectiveness of scoliosis screening. *Physiotherapy*. 1999;85(5):259–68. http://dx.doi.org/10.1016/S0031-9406(05)61440-X.
2. Klippel JH, editor. JRA diagnostic criteria *primer on the rheumatic diseases*. 13th ed. Springer; 2008. p. 142–9. http://dx.doi.org/10.1007/978-0-387-68566-3.

PART SIX

PRACTICE

28

Technical Skills for Primary-Care Doctors

The primary-care physician will need several technical skills to diagnose, stabilize, and treat orthopaedic conditions. Residents rotating through orthopaedics always ask for more opportunities to do procedures. The dictum "see one, do one, teach one" is all too true in medical education. This chapter provides some details regarding why we do things the way we do and some tips to perform these procedures safely.

Skills in the Outpatient Clinic or Office

Splinting
The application of a below-elbow splint and a below-knee splint is very commonly done after a realignment procedure in the emergency department before transferring the patient. The splint stabilizes the fracture, protects the soft tissues, and greatly increases patient comfort. Splints can be used postoperatively as well to maintain alignment while the swelling slowly decreases. The splint should be designed to last several days.

TECHNICAL CHECKLIST FOR SPLINTING

- Get help holding the limb.
- Apply adequate padding to half plaster slab.
- Apply slab as a buttress to resist potential redisplacement of the fracture (i.e., dorsal forearm in Colles'; postlateral side in typical ankle fracture).
- Leave adequate room opposite to buttress for swelling.
- Wrap smoothly but not tightly with Kling gauze. (**Avoid** tensor bandages as they tighten over time.)
- Below-knee splint extends to MT heads but not too high into popliteal fossa.
- Below-elbow splint extends to metacarpal (MC) heads but must allow easy flexion at antecubital fossa.

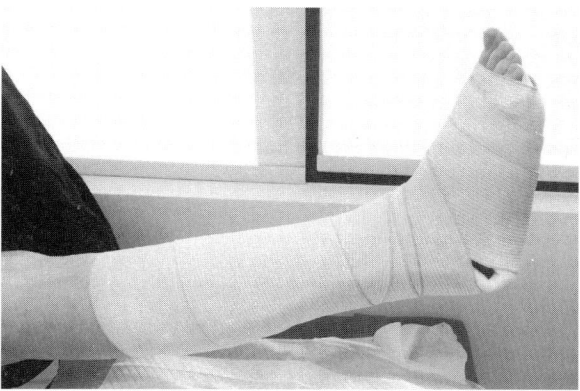

Figure 28.1 Below-knee posterior half-splint

Casting

With the advent of rigid internal fixation and removable air casts, the need to apply casts is decreasing. However, the below-elbow cast is still widely used after the initial postreduction splint has been removed in distal radius fractures. Casts are also used in ankle fractures after the swelling has decreased. Casting is still used extensively with children when compliance with air-boot wear is an issue. In addition, above-elbow and above-knee casts are still used frequently in children for the first 4–6 weeks of fracture care. They are well tolerated by children, but they should be used only occasionally with adults since they are poorly tolerated and quickly lead to stiffness.

Plaster casts are less expensive and easier to mould after closed reductions. We generally use them (or splints) until all the swelling has gone (1–2 weeks) and then convert to Fibreglass casts, which are lighter and stronger. Most casts will only last 1 month, so patients should be seen at least monthly.

TECHNICAL CHECKLIST FOR CASTING

- Get help holding the limb.
- Use adequate soft roll material.
- Roll on smoothly, not tightly.
- Pad bony prominences; avoid clumps.
- If using **plaster**, use warm water, not hot, which can scald skin under the cast.
- If using **Fibreglass**, use cold water; wear gloves.
- Cast in comfortable, functional positions with neutral alignment:
    wrist: gentle palmarflexion
    ankle: neutral dorsiflexion
    knee: 10-degree to 15-degree flexion
    elbow: 90-degree flexion

- Use three-point moulding around fracture site (distal/apex/proximal to fracture).
- Trim around thumb/antecubital fossa or toes/popliteal fossa.
- Anticipate swelling: univalve cast as required (especially Fibreglass).
- For weight bearing, use either a cast sandal or a walking knob; must be well placed and reinforced.

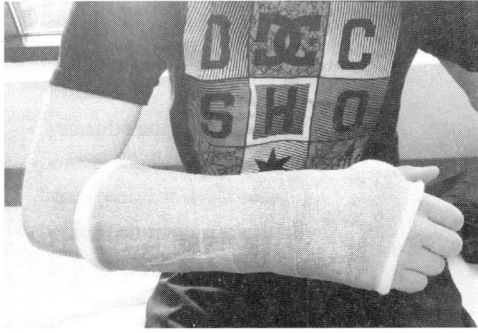

Figure 28.2 Below-elbow Fibreglass cast

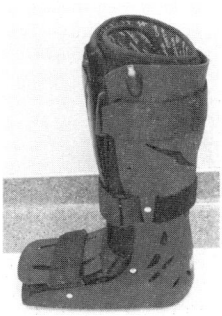

Figure 28.3 An air boot is often much simpler than a below-knee cast.

Joint and Bursa Aspiration

Joint aspirations can all be performed in the outpatient clinic or office and, with a little practice, can safely be performed by any primary-care physician. Not all joints can be aspirated in the clinic. Some are too deep or too technically challenging and should be done under fluoro in the X-ray department (or in the O.R.).

Accessible joints include the knee, shoulder (specifically the subacromial space with rotator cuff tear), lateral elbow, and bursa. Inaccessible joints include the hip, ankle, deep shoulder/glenohumeral joint (without cuff tear), and wrist.

TECHNICAL CHECKLIST FOR JOINT ASPIRATION

Knee

- Patient supine.
- Flex knee 10–15 degrees over pillow. (Quadriceps must be relaxed.)
- Use superior medial or superiolateral entry; sterile technique.
- Freeze site with local anaesthetic down to capsule using 25 g needle.
- Aspirate with 18–20 g needle. (Match the angle of the patellofemoral joint = oblique/downward.)
- No resistance if in correct space (to aspirate or inject).

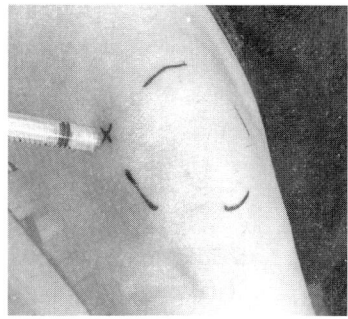

Figure 28.4 Landmarks for knee joint aspiration

Shoulder (subacromial space)

- Patient seated; arms resting on lap.
- Utilize gravity to open up interval in posteriolateral corner of acromium.
- Usually do not need to freeze skin since the joint is superficial.
- Use 25 g needle (1 cc lidocaine + 1 cc Depo-Medrol).
- True glenohumeral joint aspiration (in absence of a cuff tear) means an anterior tap is required (need fluoro).

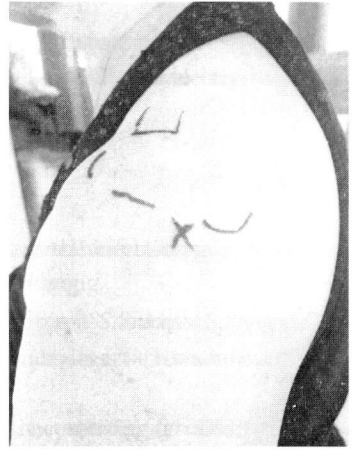

Figure 28.5 Landmarks for subacromial space injection

Elbow

- Patient supine; elbow flexed on pillow.
- Should be able to feel the effusion in the safe triangle (radial head; lateral epicondyle; olecranon).
- No freezing required; go straight in with a 22–25 g needle.
- Procedure should be relatively easy if effusion is present.

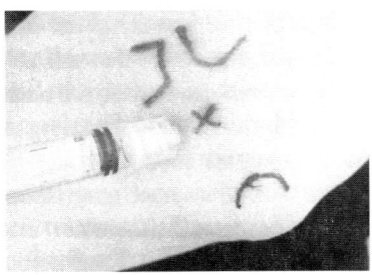

Figure 28.6 Site of elbow aspiration (safe triangle zone)

Bursa

- Superficial and commonly aspirated to relieve pressure and to rule out infection.
- Common sites include the subacromial bursa, prepatellar bursa, and olecranon bursa.

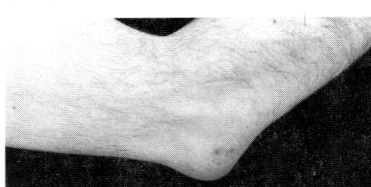

Figure 28.7 Moderate olecranon bursa enlargement

Depo-Medrol Injections

Depo-Medrol injections can be quite therapeutic for many patients, particularly the first and second injections. In general, injections should be limited to twice per year.[1] If one is in the correct interval, the injection should be relatively painless for the patient, as there should be minimal resistance. **Common joints** injected include the knee (for osteoarthritic flare-ups) and the shoulder subacromial space (for impingement syndrome).

Dorsal ganglia of the wrist and foot are common and are quite easy to aspirate and then inject. However, volar ganglions in the wrist are usually quite close to the radial artery and nerve branches and should not be routinely aspirated.

Tendonitis sites commonly injected with Depo-Medrol include lateral humeral epicondyle (tennis elbow), the first extensor compartment of the thumb (de Quervain's) and, occasionally, tendons and joints in the foot and ankle.

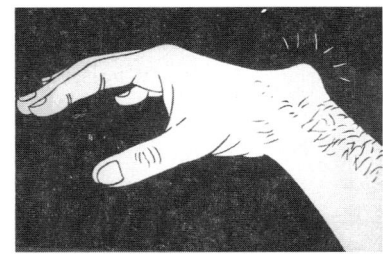

Figure 28.8 Dorsal wrist ganglion

Generally, one locates the site of maximal tenderness and then injects a 1 cc lidocaine/1 cc Depo-Medrol mixture slowly into the tendon insertion site or tendon sheath. Sometimes only a small amount of fluid can be comfortably injected.

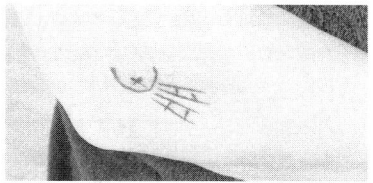

Figure 28.9 Landmarks for tennis elbow injection

Skills in the Emergency Department

Realignment Procedures in the E.R.

Realignment is not the same thing as definitive reduction. **Realignment** means correcting the gross deformity so the limb looks straighter and the pressure is relieved from the soft tissues. **Definitive reduction** means the displaced bone or joint is placed back into anatomic position, the degree to which can only be adequately assessed on X-ray. Doctors in training worry too much about reducing a fracture perfectly before it is referred on for definitive care. This anxiety is not necessary. The job of a primary-care physician is to diagnose and then treat the fracture if it can be treated in the primary-care setting, or safely transport the patient and limb for definitive care if it cannot.

Realignment takes the pressure off the soft tissues at the apex of the deformity, improves blood flow to the distal extremity, and greatly increases patient comfort. The X-ray does not need to look perfect — this is not your goal. The extremity should look better: the fingers or toes should

> Realign the extremity for the soft tissues and circulation. Do not worry about perfectly "reducing" the fracture radiographically; that is the job of the orthopaedic specialist.

"pink up" and the soft tissues should "look happier."

Common examples of injuries where realignment and splinting are highly recommended before transfer include the following:

- ankle fracture/dislocation
- tibial shaft fracture (Knee and toes should face the same direction.)
- wrist or forearm fracture
- in children: supracondylar humeral fractures

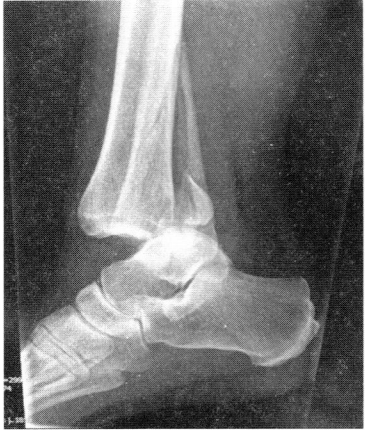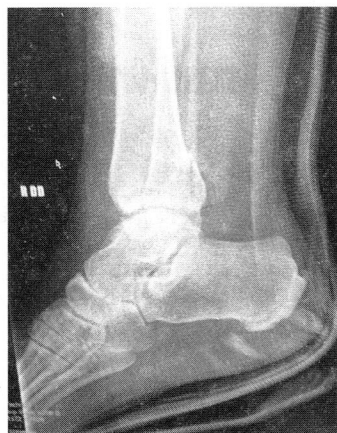

Figure 28.10 Ankle fracture/dislocation realignment (Now the patient can be safely transferred.)

Definitive Fracture Reduction in the E.R.

Certain common fractures are amenable to definitive reduction and treatment in the primary-care setting. These include the following fractures in children:

- true Colles' wrist fractures (extra-articular, dorsally angulated)
- metaphyseal and Salter II wrist fractures
- greenstick fracture in forearm
- some tibial shaft fractures

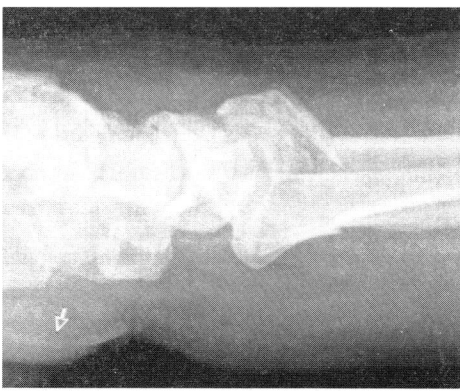

Figure 28.11 Colles' fracture of wrist with displacement

TECHNICAL CHECKLIST FOR ANAESTHETIC PREPARATION FOR COLLES' AND WRIST FRACTURE REDUCTIONS

- Get help to manage airway as required and to hold limb once reduced.
- Give adequate anaesthesia (IV sedation + local; or regional block).
- Local hematoma block (quite straightforward, but other techniques available).
- Inject about 10 cc of 2% xylocaine/no epinephrine right into dorsal fracture site. (You can usually feel the step deformity.)
- Wait 5 minutes for the anaesthetic to take effect; reduce fracture.
- Ensure adequate monitoring (IV + O^2 saturation).

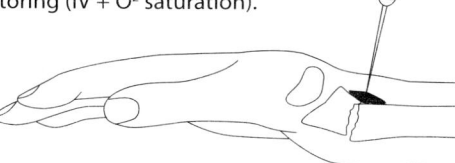

Figure 28.12 Hematoma block wrist: inject right into fracture site dorsally

TECHNICAL CHECKLIST FOR COLLES' FRACTURE REDUCTION

First X-ray, prereduction (both AP and lateral)

- Use two hands; exaggerate the deformity; distract the patient; reduce "around the corner."
- Hold reduction while splinted or casted. (Use a dorsal half-splint or a cast that is univalved volarly to allow for postreduction swelling.)

Second X-ray, postreduction

Is the reduction acceptable? Check these parameters:

- *AP X-ray:* radius length: radial styloid 1 cm longer than ulnar styloid
  - radius and ulna length equal at DRUJ?
  - wrist joint: no steps, should be perfect

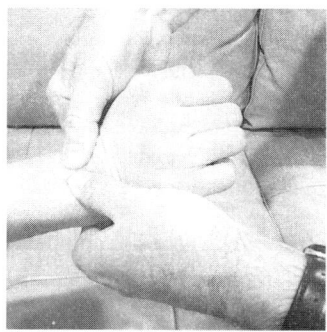

Figure 28.13 Wrist fracture reduction technique (Note how deformity is exaggerated before reducing the fracture around the corner.)

- *lateral X-ray:* joint alignment should be neutral (0 degrees) or up to 10 degrees volar (no dorsal tilt)
  - no dorsal (or volar) displacement more than 5 mm
  - minimal dorsal cortex comminution (unstable)

Reduction of Dislocations in the E.R.

Common dislocations can be definitively treated in the primary-care setting and then followed in the clinic. These always look dramatic and the patient is usually distressed, but most are quite straightforward to reduce and, thus, very gratifying for the patient and the doctor.

Choose the dislocations that can be safely done in the emergency department. The key to successful reduction is adequate muscle relaxation. To achieve this, you may have to protect the airway or bag the patient. Always have help available and make sure to get pre- and post-reduction X-rays to identify potential problems.

> The key to successful reduction is adequate muscle relaxation.

TECHNICAL CHECKLIST FOR COMMON SITES OF DISLOCATION

Shoulder
- 90% of dislocations anterior; remaining 10% more posterior than inferior
- +/– greater tuberosity fracture (unless very large)
- various techniques; "lift shoulder over glenoid rim"
    - sling compliance important if first dislocation
    - early surgery/repair of labrum in athletes?[2]

Ankle
- most ankle fractures or dislocations posteriolateral
- easy to reduce since they are so unstable

Total Hip Replacement
- usually posterior
- X-ray first to rule out implant loosening, or fracture
- for hip replacement, probably best to call orthopaedic specialist first before attempting reduction in E.R. just in case there are other concerns
- easy if recurrent dislocation; first time can be tricky

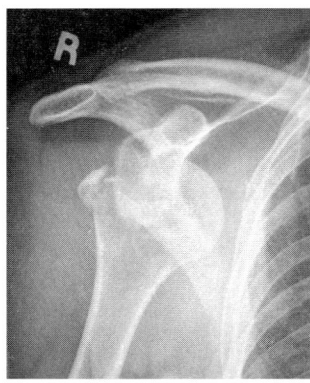

Figure 28.14 Anterior shoulder dislocation (with small greater tuberosity avulsion fracture)

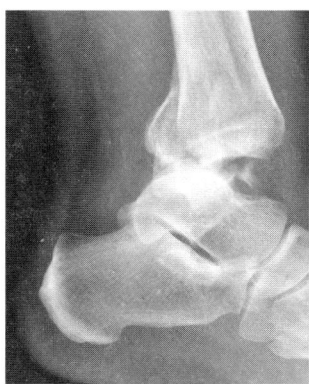

Figure 28.15 Posterior ankle fracture/dislocation

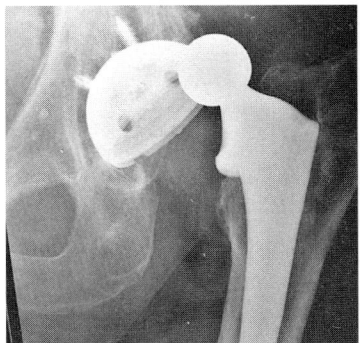

Figure 28.16 THR dislocation

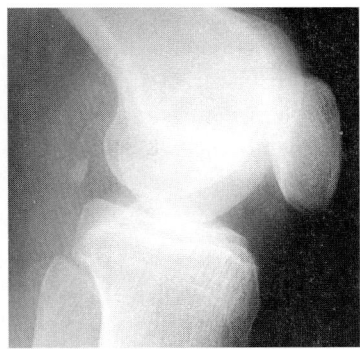

Figure 28.17 Lateral patellar dislocation; look for avulsion fractures

- distract patient; lift ball into acetabulum
- mobilize in proportion to the stability that exists; needs orthopaedic follow-up

Patellar (lateral)
- usually occurs in young girls with hyper-laxity of joints
- many reduced while positioning for X-ray
- extend knee; apply gentle medial pressure
- rule out osteochondral fractures (patellar, or lateral femoral condyle)
- may need arthroscopy

Elbow (posterior)
- high-energy injury; usually young adults
- avoid if large fracture present (other than medial epicondyle)
- use push or pull technique; be gentle
- watch for stiffness and heterotopic bone formation postreduction
- some feel NSAIDs should be used rou-tinely for 1 month[3]

Fingers and toes
- common; many reduced in the field
- ensure that no associated open fracture present
- easy unless button-holed in soft tissue (look for skin puckering)
- buddy tape to healthy digit
- watch for early stiffness (in the hand)

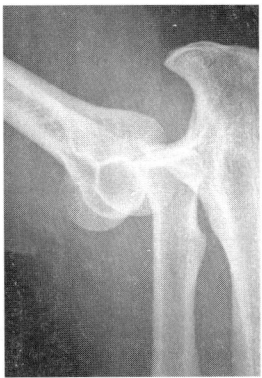

Figure 28.18 Posterior elbow dislocation

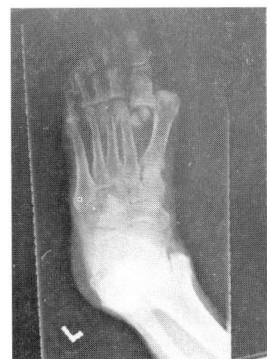

Figure 28.19 Great toe dislocation and metatarsal fractures D2 and D3

Conclusion

Many straightforward techniques can be performed by physicians in the primary-care setting, in both the elective- and emergent-care settings, to provide predictable and immediate relief of MSK symptoms for patients. The key is to know which disorders can be managed in the primary-care setting and to what degree. This takes some experience.

I always recommend family physicians in training call a senior primary-care colleague in their community when they tackle a challenging new orthopaedic injury for the first time. These colleagues can help you with your first reduction on your own or with the anaesthetic and setup at your local hospital.

Of course, the primary-care physician may also call the local orthopaedic surgeon, who can give general guidelines over the telephone. If in doubt, call someone with experience first.

REFERENCES

1. Schumacher HR, Chen LX. Injectable corticosteroids in treatment of arthritis of the knee. *Am J Med*. 2005;118(11):1208–14. http://dx.doi.org/10.1016/j.amjmed.2005.05.003. Medline:16271901

2. Jakobsen BW, Johannsen HV, Suder P, et al. Primary repair versus conservative treatment of first-time traumatic anterior dislocation of the shoulder: a randomized study with 10-year follow-up. *Arthroscopy*. 2007;23(2):118–23. http://dx.doi.org/10.1016/j.arthro.2006.11.004.

3. Hildebrand KA, Patterson SD, King GJW. Acute elbow dislocations: simple and complex. *Orthop Clin North Am*. 1999;30(1):63–79. http://dx.doi.org/10.1016/S0030-5898(05)70061-4. Medline:9882725

29

Questions Frequently Asked of Orthopaedic Surgeons

To conclude this book on a lighter note, I have collected some of the questions I have often been asked over the years by students, patients, and others regarding orthopaedics. This handy reference provides answers that probably do not appear in standard textbooks.

1. How many bones are there in the body?

I have been caught on this question before; it was the first question I was asked when I spoke about my job to my daughter's Grade 5 class. Somehow, I had missed that little detail in 13 years of study!

Adults have 206 bones (126 in the appendicular skeleton and 80 in the axial skeleton; this includes the small bones of the skull and middle ear). In children, the number is about 300 but is more difficult to determine. Some infant bones are partially cartilaginous and fuse early on while the development of growth plates (secondary centres of ossification) increases the number of bones before growth cessation.

2. How long does it take the average fracture to heal?

Obviously, this depends on the age of the patient and the *personality* of the fracture (low energy/simple or high energy/complex). On average, it takes *about 3 months* to heal most fractures. This is a good starting-point date to put on insurance forms, which frequently follow a fracture event.

3. Is there a screw loose on my X-ray?

I cannot remember how many times I have been urgently asked to see a patient who has "pain and a screw loose on the X-ray." Usually, the screw is not loose but was inserted outside the plate in interfragmentary mode (90 degrees to the fracture line).

True implant and screw loosening can occur, but usually in the context of fracture nonunion or infection. Look for a zone of radiolucency — or the "windshield wiper effect" — around the screws in these cases.

4. Why does it take so long to see an orthopaedic surgeon?

This is a very common complaint from patients (and referring doctors). Orthopaedics is an operating room, resource-based specialty, so new surgeons can be hired only when resources are available. In some places, to see a nonurgent elective patient, there has been up to a two-year wait for the initial consultation! Most orthopaedic surgeons are only in the office once or twice per week to see new elective patients. Most of their time is spent in the operating room or in the more urgent

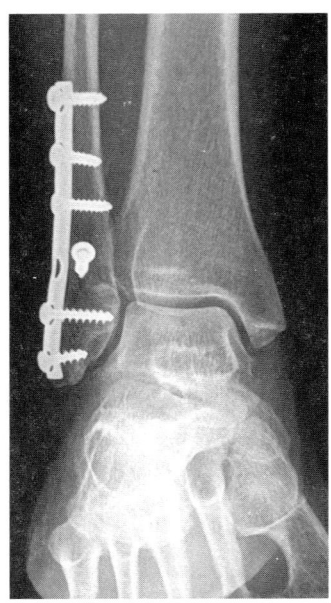

Figure 29.1 Third screw from the bottom, designed not to be in the plate, at the original operation

fracture clinic setting. However, if the referring primary-care doctor is truly concerned about a patient, he or she can always call one of us, and we will expedite the consult, if appropriate.

5. Will you accept this patient?

If the primary-care physician has examined the patient, has done a reasonable work-up, and has given treatment at the primary-care level before calling, then yes, we usually will accept care.

However, I always ask, "Where does the patient normally live?" This simple question will save a lot of grief later on, particularly if the patient has to wait one or two days to get a wrist or ankle fracture fixed at our local regional hospital. Follow-up care in the patient's hometown will be so much easier; therefore, if the patient can be comfortably splinted and is somewhat mobile, I usually recommend that he or she go to a hospital closer to home.

Conclusion

In orthopaedics, as in life, so many problems develop because of poor communication. As specialists, we often do not communicate enough with our referring family doctors. As treating physicians, we often assume our patients understand the situation and its implications, just as we do, when they are often too anxious and overwhelmed even to ask the right questions.

The practice of orthopaedics is fast paced and rewarding, with rapid improvement of damaged anatomy displayed on postoperative X-rays. The pieces of the jigsaw-puzzle, high-energy fracture can be put back together, or the hip joint destroyed by arthritis can be replaced with a shiny new prosthesis.

However, this is only the beginning. Remember the 3-month rule of recovery for most conditions? We need to remind our patients of this often and to communicate realistic expectations to them regularly. Most of our patients do get better, but orthopaedic disability can potentially be a big issue. The better we communicate with our patients, support staff, and referring doctors, the fewer disappointing outcomes we will have. Communicate, at every step of the way, and everyone wins!

Index

About the Author

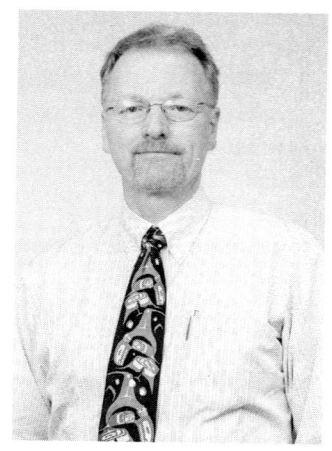

Robert Perlau was born in Edmonton, Alberta. After receiving his medical degree and family practice training from the University of Alberta, he practiced family medicine for one year in rural Alberta before starting orthopaedic specialty training at the University of Calgary, followed by one year of orthopaedic fellowship training in arthritis surgery at Harvard University in Boston, Massachusetts.

Dr. Perlau has practised general orthopaedic surgery in Red Deer, Alberta, since 1994 and has been director of orthopaedic teaching for the University of Alberta rural residency program since its inception. He is passionate about medical education and has presented his research at the Canadian Orthopaedic Association national meetings.

Dr. Perlau is currently the chief of surgery for the Red Deer Regional Hospital and Central Alberta Zone and assistant clinical professor of surgery at the University of Alberta.